JENNY

Your Diabetes
Questions Answered

Blood Sugar
101

Practical Solutions That Work
and Keep on Working

TECHNION Books

Published by Technion Books
P.O. Box 402
Turners Falls, MA 01376
technionbooks@outlook.com

ISBN-13:978-0-9647116-7-9
ISBN-10: 0-9647116-7-2

Table of Contents

Charts and Checklists

Introduction

The chances are you've picked up this book because you or someone you care about have been diagnosed with Type 2 Diabetes and you're filled with far more questions than your doctor can answer in the 15 or 20 minutes set aside for your latest appointment.

If it's been a while since you got that diagnosis, you may have started to wonder why so little of the advice you've received has made any difference. You've taken the pills your doctor prescribed, but your A1C remains stubbornly diabetic. You've tried eating the healthy diet described on the "Beat Diabetes!" flyer you were given and cut out fatty foods, but your fasting blood sugar keeps rising. You may even have joined a gym, but though you've lost a couple pounds, your toes are starting to hurt and your doctor just muttered something about early diabetic neuropathy.

Perhaps you've tried some alternative approaches and filled up your medicine cabinet with strangely named supplements that were supposed to lower your blood sugar but only lowered your bank balance. Maybe you've tried eating an alternative diet where you gave up everything you like to eat in favor of brown rice, raw fruit, and green leaves. When you burnt out on that you may have switched to an Atkins diet and eaten nothing but meat and cheese for a month, which lowered your blood sugar but made your breath stink so badly your spouse threatened to leave if you didn't give it up.

Well, welcome to the club. This kind of journey is what most people go through when they get a diabetes diagnosis. But the frustration they experience during this initial burst of enthusiasm explains why so many people give up fighting their diabetes. They just take the pills they're given, ignore their weight, and dread their doctor's appointments.

This kind of denial can actually work pretty well for a while. Until it doesn't. Feet start to go numb. The doctor mutters about your kidney function tests. The eye doctor tells you they need to see you every three months instead of just once a year.

I've been there and done quite a bit of all that myself, starting back when I was first diagnosed in 1998. But after going through years of the same kind of trial and error, burnout and denial, I got lucky and ran into some very smart people with diabetes on an online diabetes support newsgroup, alt.support.diabetes. The strategies they described, which made it possible for them to achieve impressive blood sugars, taught me that there are moderate, sustainable ways to control diabetic blood sugars that don't require us to go to extremes. My subsequent research has confirmed that these approaches are safe and will prevent diabetic complications without requiring that we give up everything that tastes good, live at the gym, or obsess about our health 24/7.

I've been a professional writer since the mid-1980s. So as I started figuring this stuff out, I wrote about it and posted what I wrote online so other people wouldn't have to waste as much time as I had on the error part of "trial and error." Those postings eventually morphed into my website, **http://bloodsugar101.com**, which I started back in 2005.

Since then, I've kept up with the research about diabetes. I've added new pages to the site whenever something important emerged and backed up the statements that appeared on the site with documentation that would let readers read the actual studies reported and draw their own conclusions.

The Blood Sugar 101 website grew so large that it became far too big for people to read all of it off of a screen. So in 2008 I turned the information stored on the site into a book, *Blood Sugar 101: What They Don't Tell You About Diabetes,* which ended up spending two whole years at the very top of the Amazon Diabetes bestseller list. Readers loved it, recommended it to friends, and gave copies as gifts to relatives.

These readers have turned *Blood Sugar 101* into a diabetes classic. It is still available in a longer, fully revised second edition, published in 2016, which is still going strong.

Why This New Book About Diabetes?

Since *Blood Sugar 101* came out, I've gotten hundreds of emails filled with questions from readers. Some, though by no means, all of those questions already were answered in Blood Sugar 101. But my correspondents seemed to have difficulty finding the answers to their questions in that book because of the way the information in it was presented.

This was understandable. Because I'm not a doctor or a trained diabetes educator, when I wrote that book I knew I couldn't expect anyone to take my advice seriously unless I backed up every point I made with references to solid, mainstream medical research. To establish that I wasn't just some off-the-wall crank, I had to go into great detail when describing the findings of the vast body of neglected mainstream medical research that supports the legitimacy of the powerful but unconventional strategy for combating diabetes that I laid out there. But that research got pretty technical at times, more technical than some of my readers were comfortable with.

So that made me think that a new book might be helpful—one that focused entirely on answering the kinds of questions my readers wrote me. This book wouldn't need to cite the research that lay behind the answers I would give, because that documentation can already be found on **bloodsugar101.com** or in the earlier book. Instead this new book would focus on troubleshooting Type 2 Diabetes. It would answer several hundred of the most pertinent questions readers had sent me over the years, dealing with them in the same way that I would have replied to them if I'd received those questions in my in-basket.

This is that book.

Some of the questions you'll find here are very basic and may repeat information you've seen elsewhere. I answer those questions so that readers who are new to the subject of Type 2 Diabetes will get the grounding they need to be able to follow the more advanced topics covered further on. But many of the questions you'll find here are those people with Type 2 Diabetes only know enough to ask years after a diagnosis, after they have tried various approaches and run into the problems that arise while trying to make them work. Those questions are rarely answered in other diabetes books currently on the market, because so few of those books are written by people who have lived with diabetes. These are questions that only a person with diabetes would think to ask—or be able to answer.

Though there is some overlap here with what you may have read in *Blood Sugar 101*, there's also quite a bit I couldn't fit into the older book. In particular, you will find much that is new in this book about how to make the most out of your relationship with your doctor. Since I wrote the first book back in 2008, that relationship has become even more difficult. Insurers now make it much tougher to get some of the prescriptions many of us need, and doctors rely a lot more on our A1C test results than they used to. These factors are making it much tougher to get the help we need to achieve the normal blood sugars that will keep us from developing the complications too many of our doctors assume are inevitable.

Over the last couple of years I've started hearing from quite a few readers who are being severely affected by these changes in the healthcare system. Though they've been very successful at lowering their blood sugars using the diet and drug regimens I described in *Blood Sugar 101* and will lay out for you in this book, some report that their doctors or insurers have decided they no longer have diabetes and have taken away the drugs that let them keep their blood sugars so normal. This poses challenges new to those of us who have spent the past decades demonstrating that the terrible complications experienced by far too many people with Type 2 Diabetes are entirely avoidable.

But they are solvable challenges, and there are a lot worse things you can hear in a doctor's office than that your blood sugar has become too normal. My hope is that the answers you'll find in this book will ensure that that is the worst message you ever will get from your own doctor.

A Few Words of Caution

This book is written for people who have been diagnosed with Type 2 Diabetes. So when I write about "diabetes" in the following pages I mean Type 2 Diabetes unless I specifically mention a different type. While people with Type 1 might find some useful information in these pages, much of what is discussed here may not be relevant to them. Type 1 Diabetes is far more difficult to manage than Type 2, and controlling it requires a different set of strategies. So this is not an appropriate book to give or recommend to someone who has just been diagnosed with Type 1 Diabetes or its adult onset form, LADA.

The questions presented here are the kinds of questions I've been sent by the many readers who have contacted me over the years. My hope is that the answers to these questions give you a lot more insight into what it takes to master Type 2 Diabetes and that they also help you get the most out of the limited time your doctor can spend with you. But it is *not* my intention to provide specific answers to the kinds of questions that only your own doctor should answer.

I don't have access to your medical records and can't answer your specific questions about your health. I may point to what the drug's label says about dosage or cite published research that highlights potential issues with a drug. But you should never rely entirely on any book for answers to questions like what specific dose of a drug you should be taking or whether a drug is safe for someone with some other medical condition you might have.

To get those answers you must consult with your personal doctor. I do occasionally point out situations where busy physicians may get dosages wrong or ignore important side effects or interactions with other drugs you are taking. If you aren't sure about something your doctor has prescribed, consult with the registered pharmacist at the pharmacy that dispenses your medications.

Along the same lines, if you are having a scary symptom that you fear might mean you are having a dangerous hypo or a heart attack put down this book and don't rely on Dr. Google. Phone your doctor's office if you have a doctor. If you don't, call an ambulance.

I had an uncle who tried to save a few bucks by waiting until Monday to call his doctor about a nasty pain he was having in his chest, because he didn't want to waste money going to the ER, since it might turn out to be nothing. It turned out to be something, and he didn't live until Monday. So if in doubt, spend the money to get that expert opinion.

Note: Whenever specific blood sugar readings are mentioned in these pages, I give them first in the units used in the United States, mg/dl and then, in curly brackets, I give the equivalent value in the mmol/L units that are used in almost every other country around the world.

Chapter One
Help! I Have Type 2 Diabetes!

I Just Got the News—What Should I Do First?

The first thing you may need to do is calm down, especially if your imagination is filling up with memories of all the awful things that happened to Aunt Maria, Grandpa Mike, or Mr. White at work, whose diabetes ruined their lives. Even the worst of today's doctors does a better job helping patients avoid those terrible outcomes than was the case even 20 years ago.

But that said, you don't want to calm down too much. Because the strong emotions you are feeling right now represent energy you can channel into doing what you have to do to ensure that diabetes never becomes more than a footnote to your life, not its theme.

It's actually helpful to feel a little bit of panic at this stage. The people I really worry about are the people who don't let their diabetes diagnoses upset them, who figure everything will be just fine if they take the pills their doctor gave them or drink more apple cider vinegar. A little terror is healthy if it gives you the energy to make some changes that are not easy, simple, or fun. It's going to take work to put diabetes in its place—a lot of it. And you will have to keep on working at it for decades. There is no easy fix for diabetes. Anyone who tells you different usually has a bottle of expensive, magical moonbeams to sell you.

Which brings me to the next thing someone just diagnosed with diabetes needs to be aware of: when it comes to your health, the glorious world of Free Enterprise is a jungle where the wallets of people with diabetes are the prey. Doctors who never got licensed to practice medicine, fraudulent supplement companies, and a whole zoo of "alternative practitioners" pay for their McMansions and country club memberships by selling miracle cures to frightened people diagnosed with chronic illnesses.

So before we begin, it's helpful to repeat to yourself this highly protective mantra: **There are no miracle cures.**

Say it to yourself a few more times and then say it again. There *are* no miracle cures. You won't cure your diabetes by eliminating all foods that start with the letter W. There is no magical plant from Southwestern Ubantuland, no healing food, no special oil, no electronic device, no yoga position, no prayer, and no cure so powerful that the medical establishment has kept it secret because if you knew about it, it would put them out of business.

There is only one real "secret" about diabetes that your doctor may not have informed you about, which is that **it's the carbs you eat that raise your blood sugar and that cutting those carbs will lower it**. But that's not much of a secret. Many thousands of people with diabetes already know it and use that powerful truth to keep themselves healthy.

But that's pretty much it as far as simple secrets go. Because diabetes isn't simple. It behaves differently from person to person. The food, drug, or exercise regimen that works for me may not work for you, and what works for you might not work for the lady down the street.

That's why real diabetes solutions can never be described in 25 words or less. No matter how well any approach has worked for someone else, you'll still have to test it out to see if it solves the riddle that is your own case of diabetes.

The point of this book is to give you the tools you need so you can test out any approach that appeals to you. It will also help you get past the many obstacles that arise when we follow even the most successful strategies for mastering our diabetes.

But these strategies *are* successful. So calm down. You're going to be okay. You're going to keep your toes and stay off dialysis. But don't calm down too much. There's work to do!

What Exactly Is "Blood Sugar?"

You were diagnosed with Type 2 Diabetes because your blood sugar was high. But what exactly does that mean? Well, for starters, the stuff your doctor calls "blood sugar" isn't the same stuff you sprinkle into your coffee. It's a simple sugar, glucose, which is unique because it's the only kind of sugar your cells can burn for energy.

Glucose is even more essential for another reason. While most of your cells can burn fats if they run out of glucose, there are cells in your brain that can't. If these glucose-burning brain cells are deprived of glucose for more than about six minutes, they die, and when they die, so do you.

How much glucose needs to be in your bloodstream to keep this from happening? Not much. The lowest blood sugar concentration at which you might still be conscious is 20 mg/dl {11.1}. That "mg/dl" means milligrams per deciliter, which is one tenth of a liter. So for you to stay alive, you need to have about two tenths of a gram of glucose dissolved in every liter of your blood. Since you have roughly five liters of blood circulating in your body, it takes only one gram of pure glucose to keep you going. That's about a quarter of a teaspoon.

If you live in a country that uses the mmol/L unit to measure glucose, it's helpful to know that one mole of glucose weighs about 180 grams, so a millimole weighs one thousandth of that, or .18 grams.

That 20 mg/dl {1.1} blood sugar concentration is the bare minimum you need to have at all times to stay alive, but it is dangerously low. That level is what doctors call "hypoglycemia," or "a hypo" for short. The very lowest blood sugar concentration considered normal is 70 mg/dl {3.9}. When you have a typically normal blood sugar concentration of 85 mg/dl {4.7}, you have just slightly less than a teaspoon of glucose dissolved in your five liters of blood.

Though you may only have one teaspoon of glucose in your blood at any given moment, it takes a lot more than one teaspoon of glucose a day to keep you functioning. That's because your cells are constantly using up the glucose in your blood and burning it to fuel their activities. So to keep your body going for a whole day you need a steady supply of glucose to replace what your cells have taken in.

That supply comes from two sources. The most important is the meals you eat and, more specifically, the starches and sugars in the foods that make up those meals. These sugars and starches are what we call "carbohydrates," or "carbs" for short. When carbs are digested all the starches turns into pure glucose and so do some of the sugars. These digested carbs are the primary source of the glucose that circulates in your blood.

But what happens when you haven't eaten for a while? That's when you draw on your other source of glucose: your liver. The liver stores a backup supply of glucose. Some of it comes from excess carbs you've eaten, but if you aren't eating carbs, your liver can also convert some of the protein you eat into glucose and store it too. During the long stretches that pass between meals and overnight, your liver releases a steady stream of that stored up glucose to keep your blood sugar from dropping below normal.

The amount of glucose in our blood fluctuates throughout the day, even in people whose blood sugars are completely normal. The graph on the next page illustrates how a normal person's blood sugar levels rise and fall throughout an entire day.

As you can see, this person's blood sugars rise to a peak about an hour after a meal or snack. Then they sink back to the fasting level a few hours after the digestion of their most recent meal is complete. When they eat a large meal, like dinner in this illustration, it takes longer for blood sugar to drop back down to it's fasting level. Snacks raise blood sugar, too. If they are eaten when a meal is still digesting they prolong the time that blood sugar stays above its fasting level. But in general, when the many, complex systems that regulate your blood sugar are all working smoothly, your blood sugar will stay pretty steady at your usual fasting blood sugar level until you eat a meal or snack.

Normal Blood Sugar Fluctuations Throughout the Day

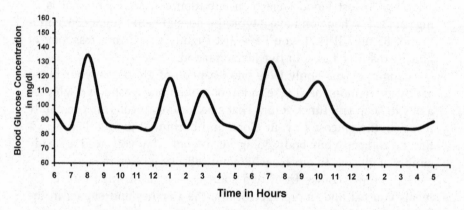

Even with these continual fluctuations, blood sugar levels in healthy fish, mammals, and healthy humans stay in a narrow range between 70 mg/dl and 140 mg/dl {3.9 and 7.8}.

Only birds and some amphibians can remain healthy when their blood sugars rise much higher than that. For example, some birds of prey may run blood sugars in the 300-400 mg/dl range {16.7 -22.2}. The record for highest blood sugar in any animal is held by hibernating wood frogs. They survive freezing solid in winter by letting their blood sugars rise as high as 100,000 mg/dl {5555.5}, which turns them, basically, into frog popsicles.

But we mammals can't withstand such high blood sugars. Blood sugars just five or six times higher than normal can kill us. Prolonged exposure to blood sugars that are only two to three times normal can destroy our hearts, kidneys, vision, nerves, and circulatory systems.

The table on the next page displays some important blood sugar levels we'll be concentrating on in the rest of the book.

Blood Sugar in Mg/dl	Blood Sugar in Mmol/L	Description
100,000	5,555.6	Blood sugar of a frozen hibernating wood frog
2,656	147.6	Highest blood sugar survived by a human
600	33.3	Blood sugar high enough to be an emergency
400	22.2	Typical highest blood sugar of a person with Type 2 Diabetes
300	16.7	Normal blood sugar for a bird of prey but damaging for a human
200	11.1	Blood sugar level at which diabetes should be diagnosed on a random blood draw
160	8.9	Highest post-meal blood sugar observed in people with normal fasting blood sugar
155	8.6	One hour glucose tolerance test blood sugar level where very early changes leading to heart disease begin
140	7.8	Two hour glucose tolerance test blood sugar level above which prediabetes is diagnosed and early complications develop
110	6.1	Fasting blood sugar associated with early complications
100	5.6	Top of the normal fasting blood sugar range above which prediabetes should be diagnosed
70	3.9	Bottom of the normal fasting blood sugar range below which blood sugars are considered hypos
40	2.2	Level at which hypos cause visual disturbances
20	1.1	Level at which consciousness starts to fade
0	0	Level that can be fatal if maintained for about six minutes

The Range of Blood Sugars Found in Nature

What is Type 2 Diabetes?

Though Type 2 Diabetes is often discussed as if it was one disease like leprosy or measles, it isn't. Everyone diagnosed with leprosy has been infected with a specific bacterium. Everyone with measles has been infected with the same virus. But there is no one cause of Type 2 Diabetes. Breakdown that happens anywhere in the complex process of blood sugar regulation can raise your blood sugars to the levels that will produce a diabetes diagnosis. So technically speaking, diabetes isn't a disease, it's a symptom, and that symptom is high blood sugar.

Doctors divide people with blood sugars high enough to be labeled "Diabetes" into two main groups. The first they diagnose as having Type 1 Diabetes. These people have abnormally high blood sugars because something has destroyed the cells in their pancreases that secrete insulin. Without insulin their cells can't burn glucose, so glucose from the meals they eat remains in their bloodstreams until its concentration rises so high it becomes life threatening.

How high is that? The Guinness World Record for highest blood sugar a person has survived is 2,656 mg/dl {147}. We aren't quite in wood frog popsicle territory at that level, but it works out to very roughly 33 teaspoons of glucose in a body's worth of blood — 33 times normal. But that's the world record. It doesn't take blood sugars anywhere near that extreme to send a person with Type 1 Diabetes to the emergency room with a condition that can be fatal if not treated immediately. Most are diagnosed when their blood sugars are somewhere between 400 mg/dl {2.22} and 600 mg/dl {33.3}. That's the level where most people with any kind of diabetes will start feeling very ill.

People with Type 1 Diabetes have completely lost the ability to secrete insulin. Usually this happens because an autoimmune attack has killed off the beta cells in their pancreas that secrete insulin. Occasionally people get diagnosed with Type 1 diabetes after surgery, a serious accident, or poisoning destroys their pancreas.

The distinguishing characteristic of Type 1 Diabetes is that anyone who has it must take supplemental insulin to stay alive. Before insulin was isolated from animal pancreases and made available to people with Type 1 Diabetes in 1922, the longest anyone had survived Type 1 Diabetes after a diagnosis was a year. And that was considered a medical miracle.

So why am I going on about Type 1 Diabetes in a book about Type 2? Because anyone whose diabetes doesn't fit a Type 1 Diabetes diagnosis is automatically diagnosed as Type 2. It's what they call a "garbage can diagnosis."

If you can survive without insulin your doctor will label you as having Type 2 Diabetes, but after you get that label they're done. No further attempt will be made to understand what is causing your abnormally high blood sugars. This remains true even though over the past decades medical research has discovered dozens—maybe even hundreds—of different and sometimes unrelated causes for the blood sugar abnormalities lumped together under the label Type 2 Diabetes.

What they all have in common, besides the fact that you can usually survive them without needing to inject insulin, is that you can have Type 2 Diabetes and be running very high blood sugars for years without noticing it. None of the "Warning Signs of Diabetes" you will find posted on health websites shows up until you have had diabetic blood sugars for years.

You may be peeing a bit more than normal, or find yourself exhausted after eating. You may keep getting urinary tract or yeast infections, too. But there are plenty of other things that could explain these symptoms. What you won't experience is the kind of dramatic crises people with Type 1 Diabetes get because most people with Type 2 Diabetes are still making enough insulin to keep them alive, just not enough to lower their blood sugars anywhere close to normal.

So if people with Type 2 Diabetes can keep on with their lives even if their blood sugars are much higher than normal, why is Type 2 Diabetes a problem? The answer is simple: Over a long period of time those non-fatal, easy to miss Type 2 high blood sugars damage your blood vessels in ways that lead to heart disease and the nasty, painful, life-altering conditions known as the classic diabetic complications.

What Exactly Is Meant by the Term "Diabetic Complications?"

The word "complications" is a euphemism, a big fat five dollar word used to make some really ugly outcomes sound less scary. The classic diabetic complications include nerve pain, blindness, lower limb amputation, and kidney failure. But doctors avoid describing these conditions in such plain language. Instead they pretty them up with less frightening, technical sounding names. Nerve pain becomes "neuropathy." (The Greek root "pathy" just means "disease.") Blindness becomes "retinopathy." Kidney failure becomes "nephropathy."

But though doctors can make the names sound less scary, they can't heal any of these conditions once they have become firmly established. So please, let the thought of complications frighten you enough that you do what it takes to ensure that you don't get them. Despite what you might have heard, that isn't all that hard to do, as you'll learn in the next couple pages.

If you're reading this at a time when you have already developed some early complications—you're in good company. About half of all people diagnosed with Type 2 Diabetes already have some early complications on the day they're first diagnosed. But that doesn't mean you're doomed. It just means that you'll have to stop putting off doing something about the high blood sugars that are causing those complications. Lowering your blood sugar back to normal or near normal levels can heal up painful nerves and improve kidney function. It will prevent amputations and keep your retinas working the way they are supposed to.

If you're impatient to know exactly how you will do this, you can skip ahead to Chapter Three.

What Causes Complications?

All the diabetic complications seem to begin after prolonged exposure to high blood sugars damages your blood vessels. These include the arteries that supply your heart and the much smaller blood vessels that supply your retinas, kidneys, and nerves.

High blood sugars make these blood vessels stiff and fragile. Over time they tend to rupture and bleed. When this happens, plaques in your coronary arteries give way and cause heart attacks, tiny capillaries in your retinas start leaking and are replaced by abnormal new ones, and the capillary systems in your kidneys stop filtering blood properly.

Nerve damage is the diabetic complication most people experience first. Like the other complications, it is caused by damaged blood vessels, in this case the tiny capillaries that supply your nerves. When your nerves don't get enough oxygen they start to die, starting from your toes up. This nerve damage hurts for a while. Then as it progresses your nerves die off and become numb. This may feel a bit better but dead nerves make you more prone to infections.

Amputations are among the most feared diabetic complications. Two factors work together to make them happen. The first is a side effect of your nerves having been destroyed by high blood sugars. That's because your nerves do much more than let you know something hurts. They also notify the immune system when tissue is damaged or when you are under bacterial attack. Dead nerves no longer can do this, so invading microorganisms can feast on your flesh undisturbed, because your immune system is no longer getting the message that your defenses have been breached.

Even if your immune system does become aware that you are fighting off an invader, your sugar-clogged, damaged blood vessels make it hard for immune cells to reach the site of the infection. This is why people who have had very high diabetic blood sugars for decades end up suffering the incurable infections and gangrene that force doctors to amputate their lower limbs.

Several other conditions that often occur a while before someone is diagnosed with Type 2 Diabetes are also caused by damage to blood vessels. These include tendon problems like frozen shoulder and carpal tunnel syndrome, and, some doctors believe, vertebral disc disease. That's because tendons and discs have a scanty blood supply at the best of times, so they are among the tissues that are the first to be affected when the smallest blood vessels begin to experience damage.

Does An Underlying Condition Cause Complications?

Many people have told me their doctors insist it isn't just high blood sugars that cause diabetic complications and heart disease but that there is some underlying condition people with Type 2 Diabetes have that makes complications inevitable. I've heard the same story from my own doctors. If it really were true, it would be futile to try to lower our blood sugars to prevent complications. But it isn't.

Many doctors seem to think that the underlying condition that makes complications inevitable is the insulin resistance they also believe is the main cause of Type 2 Diabetes. But people with Type 1 Diabetes get heart disease and all the rest of the classic diabetic complications despite having no insulin resistance at all.

Others point to obesity and the inflamed fat that often accompanies it as the underlying condition that causes diabetic complications. But again, that wouldn't be a factor for people with Type 1 Diabetes who tend to be thin. Yet those thin, insulin sensitive Type 1s not only get heart disease and all the identical classic diabetes complications that obese people with Type 2 get—they get them at younger ages.

The only thing people with both types of diabetes have in common is that they all spend many hours each day with extremely high blood sugars. So it seems logical that exposure to high blood sugars is enough to explain why people with any form of diabetes get heart disease and all the classic diabetic complications.

What Blood Sugar Levels Cause Complications?

If it's high blood sugars and only high blood sugars that cause complications, the obvious question to ask is, "How high?" I asked this question myself 12 years ago and then spent many months reading research published in medical journals to see if the data available there could point to a clear cut answer.

It turned out it did. Studies performed by researchers all over the world, who investigated the impact of specific blood sugar levels on individual cells, mice, rats, and large groups of humans all pointed to a very narrow range of blood sugars as being where trouble started. Not only that, but the toxic levels they identified turned out to be in the range doctors currently label "prediabetic."

This explains why so many people with supposedly well-controlled diabetes get heart disease, nerve damage, and all the rest of the classic complications. This "prediabetic" blood sugar range is much lower than the level doctors tell their Type 2 Diabetes patients to aim for.

If you're interested in the details, you can read about the studies that pinpointed the blood sugar levels that lead to complications on these two Blood Sugar 101 web pages: "Research Connecting Blood Sugar Level with Organ Damage" which you'll find at **http://bloodsugar101.com/14045678.php** and "Post-Meal Blood Sugars and High Normal A1cs Predict Heart Attack" which you'll find at **http://www.bloodsugar101.com/15945839.php**.

If you're not into reading medical research papers here's the short version: The very early changes in our blood vessels that eventually lead to heart disease start to happen when people's blood sugars rise over 155 mg/dl {8.6} *one hour* after the start of a glucose tolerance test. (You can read more about this test on Page 23.)

Studies of large populations where blood sugars were estimated using the A1C test, which you can read more about on Page 28, came up with a similar finding: People with or *without* diabetes whose A1Cs remain under F.0% have the very lowest risk of having a heart attack.

This is true no matter what they weigh or what their cholesterol levels might be. That 5% A1C supposedly translates to an average blood sugar of 98 mg/dl. {5.4}.

For each additional 1.0% rise in A1C in these large population studies the risk of a heart attack doubles though it still remains quite low until the A1C rises above 6.0%. That 6.0% A1C can be achieved by having blood sugars that average 126 mg/dl {7.0}. Since that is the average, people with a 6.0% A1C are almost certainly experiencing blood sugar fluctuations that are likely to rise well over the 155 mg/dl {8.6} level that other research points to as being the threshold over which arterial changes leading to early heart disease begin.

The level at which the rest of the diabetic complications start to become visible is only a little bit higher. They start showing up in people whose blood sugars remain over 140 mg/dl {7.8} *two hours* after the start of a glucose tolerance test.

This is a longer period of time than the *one hour* reading we just saw applies to heart disease. To have a blood sugar of 140 mg/dl two hours after consuming glucose, you would have to have had either a much higher blood sugar at one hour into the test or one modestly higher that took a long time to come down. Unfortunately, we don't have evidence about what the peak was that people experienced while taking these glucose tolerance tests, only that two hours after they started, their blood sugar was still over 140 mg/dl {7.8}.

But what you should take away from this is that 140 mg/dl is the "magic number" when it comes to developing complications. It shows up as a critical threshold in studies of diabetic neuropathy (nerve pain), nephropathy (kidney disease), and retinopathy (eye damage). Blood sugars that stay over this level two hours after a glucose challenge — and probably after a meal — are doing damage. You should also keep in mind that doctors define that 140 mg/dl {7.8} blood sugar level as being only "prediabetic" and are not aware of how damaging they can be.

In the case of diabetic kidney disease, there is one more blood sugar factor that plays a part. Blood sugars that surge up and down steeply turn out to be worse for you than blood sugars, even high ones, that remain relatively flat. Something about large changes in blood sugar concentration seems to damage our kidneys.

There are a few other unpleasant conditions that don't usually make it onto the list of diabetic complications that also become more frequent when people's blood sugar are over 140 mg/dl {7.8} two hours after consuming glucose. The most notable are vertebral disc degeneration and tendon problems including frozen shoulder, carpal tunnel syndrome, and piriformis syndrome.

This research suggests very strongly that there is no mysterious underlying condition that causes diabetic complications. It's the high blood sugars that do it and they start doing it at those prediabetic levels too many doctors ignore.

If the thought of getting your blood sugar down to anything remotely near normal fills you with dread because your readings now are so much higher, don't despair. Lots of us have done it and have kept on doing it for a decade or longer. You can read many fascinating reports submitted by people who have made remarkable changes to their blood sugars on the Blood Sugar 101 web page "The 5% Club: They Normalized Their Diabetic Blood Sugars and So Can You!" which you'll find   at **http://www.bloodsugar101.com/16535158.php.** There you will see that people with A1Cs approaching 17% have been able to get their blood sugar down to levels their doctors considered normal in only a few months. Not only that, many have kept on doing it year after year.

You can do it too!

Why Did My Relative Lose a Limb and Go on Dialysis?

It is hard for me to think about the extraordinarily poor care people with diabetes received a mere generation ago without being overcome with rage.

Doctors ordered their patients to eat high carbohydrate/low fat diets that made it impossible for them to control their blood sugars and left them ravenously hungry. When that diet didn't work, they were put on either insulin or insulin-stimulating oral drugs. These drugs made them even hungrier while forcing them to eat carbs all day long in order to avoid having severe hypoglycemic attacks.

Hypos were a constant concern because people with Type 2 Diabetes had no idea how high their blood sugars were most of the time. Until the mid-1990s they were rarely given blood sugar meters. The first time I ever saw a meter was in 1985, during my *second* diabetic pregnancy—after I was wheeled into the delivery suite. Like everyone else with Type 2 back then, the only blood sugar tests I ever had were the ones taken when I visited the lab before a doctor's visit. Even then, I had no idea how high my blood sugars were. All I was told was that they were diabetic. It didn't occur to me to ask for more details.

Your older relatives not only couldn't lower their diabetic blood sugars—since they rarely knew what they were—they were instructed not to. Because of the fear of hypos, conscientious doctors urged their patients to keep their blood sugars safely high. A1Cs of 9% or 10% were encouraged. It wasn't until 1992 that a large study proved that lowering A1Cs to what at the time was considered a very low level— 7.0%--made a huge difference in how many patients developed the most serious forms of all the diabetic complications.

So, this explains why, as recently as the 1990s, so many people with diabetes of both types lost limbs, went blind, and had their kidneys fail. Many more didn't even live long enough to develop these classic diabetic complications, because their diabetic heart disease killed them first.

But diabetes care today is far better. You are no longer dependent on a semi-annual visit with your doctor for information about how your blood sugar is behaving. You can buy your own meter and strips at a drug store or order them online. Most insurance plans will cover testing supplies if your doctor orders them, and most doctors will prescribe them if you ask for them.

The low fat mania is over, too. Patients are no longer forced to eat fat-phobic diets so rich is carbohydrate that they push blood sugars up to levels no drug can control. Nor are we told to eat blocks of artificially colored, artery-clogging trans fat instead of butter. Excellent research has proven that diets that lower blood sugar by limiting how much carbohydrate we eat are safe and that dairy fats are not only safe but are a lot healthier than the highly processed vegetable oils that were considered healthy a generation ago. Even the American Diabetes Association (ADA) has grudgingly admitted that there is no reason people with diabetes can't safely eat a low carb diet if they want to.

So the limitations that made it so easy for earlier generations to suffer so terribly from diabetes are largely gone. You are so much luckier than your elders. Make the most of it!

How Long Does It Take to Go Blind or Lose a Foot?

It takes at least a decade of exposure to damagingly high blood sugars to produce full-fledged diabetic complications. By full-fledged complications I mean the state where your feet are numb, infections start healing slowly, your kidneys are leaking protein, and the blood vessels in your eyes are growing in abnormal patterns.

These changes are most likely to happen when your A1C has been above 8% for many years. They may still happen, perhaps a bit more slowly, when you keep your A1C closer to the 7.0% doctors label "good control." That is more likely to be the case if you have achieved that 7.0% A1C while having post-meal blood sugar spikes that rise over the middle 200s {11.4} after most meals.

But even if you have been living with very high blood sugars for a while, there is no reason to panic. Unless you have let your blood sugar stay at extremely high levels for a decade, it will take several more years to get to the point where you end up on dialysis or lose a toe.

If you start working on getting your blood sugar back down to a safer level right now, much of this damage will heal up. Your kidney function can improve. Your nerves will grow back, and further deterioration in your retinas can be halted.

So get that excess glucose out of your bloodstream and take the fear out of your future!

Do I Really Have Diabetes?

I hear from a lot of people who wonder if symptoms they are experiencing are being caused by undiagnosed diabetes. So let's take a moment to review how diabetes is diagnosed. The tests and the results that will lead to a diabetes diagnosis are listed in the table below.

No matter what symptoms you have, or what blood sugar readings you see after eating, no doctor will diagnose you with any form of diabetes unless at least one of your blood tests comes in above these diagnostic levels.

Test	Normal	Prediabetes	Diabetes
Fasting Plasma Glucose	70-99 mg/dl 3.9-5.5 mmol/L	100-125 mg/dl 5.6-6.9 mmol/L	Over 125 mg/dl Over 6.9 mmol/L
Random Blood Glucose			Over199 mg/dl Over 11.1 mmol/L
A1c	4.7-5.6%	5-7%-6.5%	Over 6.4%
Glucose Tolerance Test 2 hr	Under 140 mg/dl Under 7.8 mmol/L	140-199 mg/dl 7.8-11.0 mmol/L	Over 199 mg/dl Over 11.0 mmol/L

The Tests Doctors Use to Diagnose Diabetes

The fasting plasma glucose test, sometimes called a fasting blood sugar test, measures how high your blood sugar is when you have gone for 12 hours without eating. It's the test doctors usually use to screen for diabetes, since it is included in the comprehensive metabolic panel, which is a group of tests performed to see how your blood sugar, liver, kidneys, and electrolytes are doing.

The fasting plasma glucose test is often the very last test to register a diabetic value. Many of us go years with our blood sugars rising into the diabetic range after each meal without ever seeing a diabetic fasting plasma glucose test result.

The official document that lays out how diabetes should be diagnosed states that repeated readings over 199 mg/dl {11.1} should also lead to a diagnosis of diabetes. That document can be read at **http://care.diabetesjournals.org/content/33/Supplement_1/S62.** But few family doctors seem aware of this. So they rarely order a blood glucose test that would measure how high your blood sugars rise after eating.

The other test doctors commonly use to determine if you have diabetes is the AIC test. Until very recently, the ADA cautioned doctors not to use this test to screen for diabetes because it's not very accurate. But then cheap A1C test kits came on the market. Since doctors can administer these tests in their offices and get an instant result—and bill for the testing—the A1C test is now being used much more frequently.

The A1C test result is supposed to reflect what your average blood sugar has been over the past three months. Because this average is affected by how high your blood sugars rise after you eat, it should, in theory, do a better job of screening than the fasting plasma glucose test. But it often doesn't for reasons discussed on Page 28.

Current guidelines say that you should be diagnosed with diabetes if your A1C reading is 6.5% or higher. (This appears to has been recently revised downward from 7.0%.) A positive test should be repeated because the test can be so inaccurate. How inaccurate? One study of several different A1C test kits sold to physicians' found that a reading of 7.0% on one test kit might be a 6.5% or a 7.5% if you were tested with a different test kit.

In rare cases, doctors diagnose diabetes with glucose tolerance test. This is considered the most accurate test and is usually used in situations where it is essential that the diagnosis be correct, for example, if you are pregnant or if you are hoping to donate a kidney. This is a more complex, time-consuming test.

How it works is this: First a fasting blood sample is taken. Then you drink a big glass of glucose mixed in water. Usually the test uses 70 grams of glucose, which is about as much glucose as you'd get after digesting a large bagel. Then you sit and wait until your blood is drawn one and two hours later. Sometimes a doctor will order a version of the glucose tolerance test where your insulin levels are also measured. This is done to see if you are producing insulin and if so, how much.

If your blood sugar is over 200 mg/dl {11.1} two hours after you start a glucose tolerance test, you will be diagnosed with diabetes. If it is over 140 mg/dl {7.8} you will be told you have prediabetes.

Sometimes people will have a normal or high reading at one hour followed by a very low reading after the second hour of the test. Low here means under 70 mg/dl {3.9}. If this happens, you may be told you have reactive hypoglycemia.

Even if you have been seeing many readings over 200 mg/dl at home when you've tested your blood sugars after eating, you may still register a non-diabetic value two hours into a glucose tolerance test. This is because the pure glucose you suck down during the test hits your blood much faster than does the glucose that comes from foods you have to digest. So people who experience blood sugar spikes into the mid 200 range {around 13.9} when they eat meals may find that during a glucose tolerance test their blood sugar shoots up within 15 minutes — the time it takes glucose to reach the bloodstream — reaches a very fast peak, and then drops below the diabetic range an hour or an hour and a half later. Since only the two hour value is used to diagnose diabetes, when this happens you will be told you only have prediabetes.

If your test results don't reach any of these diagnostic levels, as far as your doctor is concerned, you don't have diabetes.

What Makes Those Blood Sugar Levels Diabetic?

One of the weirder things about diabetes is that if your fasting blood glucose comes in at 126 mg/dl {7.0} you will be told you are diabetic, but if it is only 125 mg/dl, you're not. The same is true of those nonfasting post-meal cutoffs. At 199 mg/dl you're considered "prediabetic," a diagnosis most doctors ignore. At 200, you're suddenly diabetic. One mg/dl is a tiny amount of glucose. So what has changed when you cross over that diagnostic boundary?

The answer is, "Nothing." The definition of what exactly makes a person diabetic is entirely arbitrary.

As I explained above, diabetes is really a symptom—high blood sugar— not a disease. Blood sugars rise slowly and gradually over a long period of time without anything obvious happening to tell a doctor that a person now has diabetes. It's not like one day your liver turns green or you grow a huge zit on your pancreas. Eventually those high blood sugars will damage your nerves, kidneys and retinas, but it's hard to predict when.

Doctors struggled for years to determine what blood sugar level to use to diagnose people with diabetes before high blood sugars had caused irreversible damage but they never came up with a definition everyone in the medical community could agree on.

Then, in 1978, the ADA convened a committee of experts who were tasked with defining specific blood sugar levels that would henceforth be used by all doctors to diagnose diabetes. The levels they chose were considerably higher than those many doctors had been using before the committee met. They'd been diagnosing diabetes when glucose tolerance test two hour readings were between 160 and 180 mg/dl {8.9 and 10}. But the ADA's committee chose to set a much higher diagnostic cutoff.

Their reasoning was that diagnosing patients with diabetes when their blood sugars were too low to cause complications wasn't good for them. An early diagnosis could threaten their ability to get insurance at a point in the progression of diabetes where doctors had no treatments to offer them. So the ADA's experts decided to diagnose diabetes only when a person's blood sugars had risen to the level they believed was just slightly lower than the point at which diabetic eye damage begins to occur. Based on the data available in 1978, they decided this level was 200 mg/dl {11.1.}

This made sense at the time. Diet wasn't going to help these people, as it was believed that the only safe diet for people with diabetes was the low fat, low protein diet, very high in carbohydrates that pushes blood sugars way up. The only drugs available to treat Type 2 Diabetes were all capable of causing dangerous hypos and couldn't be prescribed safely until people's blood sugars were well over that 200 mg/dl {11.1} level.

But things have changed a lot since then. We have much safer drugs, some of which are at their most effective when they are prescribed long before people's blood sugars rise to the levels the committee defined as diabetic. We have home blood sugar meters to warn us if a drug is pushing our blood sugar too low.

In addition, high quality medical research has established that the 1978 committee was wrong. Diabetic retinal changes start occurring at blood sugar levels *far lower* than 200 mg/dl {11.1}. Indeed, as we've seen, research has established that *all* the so-called diabetic complications begin to develop when people's blood sugars are only rising over 140 mg/dl {7.8}, into the range the ADA committee labeled "prediabetic."

You'd think all this would have motivated the ADA to redefine what blood sugar levels really are diabetic, so that people could be diagnosed before those "prediabetic" blood sugars started rotting out their blood vessels. But you'd be wrong.

In 1998 the ADA convened another panel of experts to review their diagnostic criteria. They decided that those 1978 diagnostic criteria had became so universally applied in medical research that it would be too disruptive to *researchers* to change them. The disruptions that early complications might cause to people who actually had diabetes didn't get discussed, but this should be no surprise. The ADA has always been about supporting the needs of those who profit from diabetes—like drug companies and academic researchers—not those who actually have it.

The 1998 committee made only a small, cosmetic change to the criteria, perhaps to justify their ADA paychecks. They lowered the *fasting plasma glucose* level used to diagnose diabetes. But if you'll recall, this is that same fasting glucose value that stays normal for many people years after their post-meal blood sugars have already started to cause early diabetic complications. Lowering the fasting diagnostic standard did lead to slightly earlier diagnoses but still left a huge number of people with undetected high blood sugars elevated enough to damage their organs. Subsequent research determined that these people whose diagnoses were missed tended to be female or people of color.

Even now, almost 20 years after the 1998 committee met, the rest of the 1978 diagnostic criteria are still intact, even though 40 years have passed since they were set too high based on scanty research and a desire to keep people from being diagnosed "too early."

People are still being diagnosed with diabetes only when their blood sugar has spent years rising well over 200 mg/dl {11.1} after meals, though researchers have proved conclusively that this level is high enough to cause heart disease and all the classic diabetic complications.

If you are reading this somewhere that isn't the United States you may be thinking, "Why should I care what some *American* Diabetes Association defined as diabetes?" The answer is, because the World Health Organization and just about every other organization that defines diagnostic standards worldwide just copies whatever guidelines the ADA has given their blessing to.

If you are interested in learning the whole, fascinating story about how these diagnostic cutoffs were set, which is much longer than I can go into here, you can read it online on the web page "Misdiagnosis by Design - The Story Behind the ADA Diagnostic Criteria," which you can find at **http://www.bloodsugar101.com/14046782.ph**p.

What Really Is a Normal Blood Sugar Level?

Now that you've learned about the relationship of blood sugar levels and diabetic complications and seen how modestly elevated blood sugar can further damage your beta cells and make it even harder to control your blood sugar, you may wonder what blood sugar levels really are normal.

But defining normal isn't as simple as it seems. The ADA tells you that anyone whose blood sugar is under 140 mg/d {7.8} two hours after consuming a big dose of glucose is normal. But when scientists measure the blood sugar of lots of normal people, they see far lower values.

Many of us with diabetes would be happy to settle for blood sugars that while perhaps not completely normal are low enough to prevent complications or, worst case, cause them to develop at a rate so slow that we can die at an advanced age with only the mildest symptoms.

The table below summarizes three different approaches to defining "normal blood sugars."

	CGMS Normal	5% Club Normal	To Avoid Complications
1 Hr after meal	120 mg/dl 6.7 mmol/L	Under 140 mg/dl 7.8 mmol/L	Under 155 mg/dl 8.6 mmol/L
2 Hrs after Meal	85 mg/dl 4.7 mmol/L	Under 120 mg/dl 6.7 mmol/L	Under 140 mg/dl 7.8 mmol/L
A1c Test	4.3% - 5.4%	5.0 - 5.9%	5.0 - 5.9%
Fasting Blood Sugar	85 mg/dl 4.7 mmol/L	Under 110 mg/dl 6.1 mmol/L	

Normal and Safe Blood Sugars

The first column shows what studies have found to be the average blood sugar when people with normal fasting blood sugars wore a Continuous Glucose Monitor System (CGMS) all day that measured their blood sugar every few minutes. The highest values seen after meals in this group of normal people ranged from 90 to 160 mg/dl {5 to 8.9} about an hour after eating.

Over the second hour after eating, these normal people's blood sugar fell back into the range between 120 mg/dl {6.6} and 60 mg/dl {3.3}. That last value is hypoglycemic, which suggests some of these people had reactive hypoglycemia (discussed further on page 45) and were beginning to lose the ability to secrete insulin normally. This casts some suspicion on how normal the 160 mg/dl high some of these people attained at one hour really was.

The second column shows the values that the people active in the alt.support.diabetes newsgroup who called themselves "The 5% Club" determined to be normal values back in the early 2000s. They drew this conclusion based on numbers that had been published on the Joslin Diabetes website at that time, These are the blood sugar levels many of us who were active on the newsgroup in its heyday have been working on maintaining since then. If you define "normal" as "not getting diabetic complications," our experience suggests they work quite well.

The final column shows the blood sugar levels that appear to be safe based on the research I compiled that connects blood sugar levels with complications which we discussed earlier.

What Is a Normal A1C?

It's much tougher to determine what a truly normal A1C reading might be than it is to figure out what is normal with direct measurements of plasma glucose. The A1C is a much less accurate test. That's because it doesn't actually measure your blood glucose levels. Instead it measures what percentage of your hemoglobin—the protein that carries oxygen in your blood—is of a specific type, hemoglobin A1c. This form of hemoglobin has had glucose become permanently bonded to it. The other kinds of hemoglobin you have, A1b, A1a1, and A1a2 don't bond to glucose. The percentage of your hemoglobin proteins that are the A1c variant can be used to estimate how high your blood sugar has been over the past three months.

This estimate rests on two assumptions. One is that the higher your blood sugar has been over the life of a red blood cell, the more glucose will have bonded to its hemoglobin and turned it into the A1c form. The other assumption is that your red blood cells live for three months. These assumptions are there because the correlation between the A1C test result and a person's actual blood sugar levels was determined by studying the *average* values in large groups of people.

But that's a lot of assumptions, so the estimate the A1C test provides is only valid if your hemoglobin proteins collect glucose at a completely average rate and your red blood cells live the average life of such a cell, which is three months. If you have any slight abnormality in the shape of your hemoglobin proteins that affects their ability to bond to glucose or if the lifespan of your red blood cells is shorter or longer than average, the A1C test will give a faulty estimate of what your average blood sugar levels have been.

Plenty of things can make just that happen. For example, if you have anemia you will get misleading A1C test results, but the direction in which the test will be wrong depends on the specific *kind* of anemia you have. If you have iron-deficiency anemia, your A1C test result will be much *higher* than it should be based on your actual blood sugar readings. If you then take iron supplements to address your iron-deficiency anemia, your A1C will drop. But don't try to lower your A1C by taking iron unless you have been diagnosed with iron-deficiency anemia. Too much iron can damage your beta cells and worsen your diabetes.

The story is very different if you have what is called hemolytic anemia. With this kind of anemia something is causing your red blood cells to die faster than usual. If that is happening, your A1C test will give a misleadingly *low* reading.

This explains why people carrying the sickle cell trait or the gene for thalassemia that is found in people of Mediterranean heritage or whose families are from Southeast Asia should be alert to the possibility that the A1C test results they get are misleading. The A1C test may also be inaccurate if you have kidney failure, extremely high triglycerides in your blood, liver disease, or are a heavy drinker.

Because very few of us have red blood cells that are completely average, it's likely your A1C test results will always be higher or lower than what you'd expect based on measuring your blood sugars at home with a meter. This makes it tough to say what would be a normal A1C test value for you. While we do know how the *average* A1C test values correlated with the likelihood of having heart disease in studies of thousands people, we don't know if *your* A1C test reflects the same actual blood sugar level over the past three months as that *average* A1C did.

So keep your eye on your actual post-meal blood sugars, which you can test at home, and don't worry about the A1C if it comes in higher than your actual readings would predict. Though the A1C is easy to administer, and hence a favorite among doctors, heart disease is the only diabetic complication where there is a strong relationship between the A1C test value and outcomes, and that is only when analyzing large groups of people and dealing solely with averages.

Studies of the relationship between A1C results and rest of the classic diabetic complications have found that the A1C is *not* useful for predicting their occurrence. People can have identical 7.0% A1Cs but have very different amounts of diabetic nerve pain and kidney disease. That's because you can achieve the same A1C by keeping your blood sugar within a very narrow range centered on the A1C-predicted average level or by running blood sugars that rise extremely high for a few hours and then plunge very low. That kind of roller coaster pattern is much more likely to produce the classic diabetic complications than the flatter one.

Why Do You and Dr. Bernstein Disagree About Normal Blood Sugars and Targets?

I have immense respect for Dr. Richard K. Bernstein. Everyone in the world who has diabetes today owes him a huge debt of gratitude for pioneering the use of the blood sugar meter and teaching the world that the secret to long lasting health for people with diabetes was to achieve normal blood sugars.

Where I have parted ways with him is in the definition of what a normal blood sugar really is, and based on that, what are appropriate blood sugar targets for people with diabetes to aim for. There is nothing wrong with shooting for the extremely low blood sugar targets that Dr. Bernstein advocates. If you can reach them there's no doubt that you will have excellent health.

The problem is that most people can't reach those levels even when eating extremely stringent diets. Dr. Bernstein assumes that if you can't reach those numbers with diet alone, you can use fast-acting insulin at mealtimes to do it. But with what insulin costs nowadays insurers are balking at covering it unless a person's A1C is very high. Doctors are less likely to prescribe insulin now unless all the new, potentially dangerous, oral drugs have been tried first. Even with fast-acting insulin it can be tough to get our blood sugar down into the 80s {4.4} he recommends without risking serious hypos.

The other problem is that very few people can eat the extremely low carbohydrate diet Dr. Bernstein insists is necessary without burning out, and as I explained earlier, burnout has very bad health consequences.

The reason I felt able to diverge from Dr. Bernstein's dietary advice is that the research I did to document what blood sugar levels cause complications supports the idea the levels Dr. Bernstein defines as "normal" in his book are much lower than those found in normal people with normal health. Dr. Bernstein himself graciously reviewed my Blood Sugar 101 book and explained that he had not had the time, as a practicing physician, to review the reams of research I'd made my way through, and that he found it very interesting.

So that is why I don't tell people, as he does, that all normal people have blood sugars that never rise above 83 mg/dl. The data contradict that. And the data also are compelling that blood sugars that spend most of the day under 140 mg/dl are enough to prevent diabetic complications and heart disease.

Does Type 2 Diabetes Always Get Worse?

I have seen it stated in the writings of quite a few medical professionals that because of the underlying mechanisms that cause Type 2 Diabetes, people who have it always get worse.

It isn't true. But this widely held belief explains why so many doctors save their energy for treating patients with other conditions where they believe that their efforts might be better rewarded.

The irony is that it is precisely because most doctors don't put much energy into helping their patients with Type 2 Diabetes achieve normal blood sugars that their patients deteriorate.

But the reason that people with Type 2 Diabetes deteriorate has nothing to do with any underlying disease process. It happens because doctors around the world follow the treatment guidelines set by the ADA which keep the blood sugars of people with diabetes at levels high enough to kill off their remaining beta cells.

Though it is never discussed as being a diabetic complication, perhaps the most damaging effect of high blood sugars is that they kill our insulin-secreting beta cells. So high blood sugars beget even higher blood sugars, which is what leads to the slow deterioration so many doctors believe to be inevitable. It shouldn't surprise you to learn that the blood sugar levels at which beta cells start suffering from this "glucose toxicity" are the same levels that cause the classic complications. Beta cells start dying off when blood sugars spend many hours each day over that 140 mg/dl {7.8} threshold. This probably explains why most people with Type 2 Diabetes have already lost 40 to 50% of their beta cells, if not more, by the time they receive an official diagnosis, since as we have seen, this is a prediabetic blood sugar level that most doctors barely consider worth mentioning.

Obviously, if you keep your blood sugars at the 7.4% A1C that the ADA defines as "excellent control" you're going to keep on killing off your beta cells. That 7.4% A1C corresponds to an average blood sugar of 166 mg/dl {9.2}. This is well over that 140 mg/dl {7.8} level where glucose toxicity starts killing them.

The good news is that, just as is the case for the classic diabetic complications, if you drop your blood sugars below that toxic level, your remaining cells should stay alive and secreting for many more years.

But a doctor who tells you that all people with Type 2 Diabetes will deteriorate is a doctor who has just told you that the care they give their patients is not good enough. If that describes yours, it would be helpful to find yourself a new doctor who is willing to support you in getting the better control that can restore you to normal health.

If you can't find a doctor like that, don't despair. Very few of us who have been active in the online diabetes community for decades have ever had any but the most minimal support from our doctors. Some of us have had to fight our doctors every step of the way, just to get a prescription for a meter or strips. Lots of us had to sit while doctors yelled at us that our low carb diets would give us fatal heart attacks, since it was suicide to eat butter instead of trans fat-filled margarine. We still managed to end up okay, and so will you, as long as you do the work it takes to keep your blood sugar below the level that kills off your beta cells.

Will Diabetes Really Shorten My Life by a Decade?

You will often read scary headlines like a recent one that claimed some study had proven that diabetes shortens people's lifespan by a decade.

When you see such a headline, remember that by "people with diabetes" researchers mean people with diabetes whose A1Cs average 7.0% or higher, who dutifully eat diets low in fat and high in so-called "healthy whole grains," starchy vegetables, and sugary fruits.

Their A1Cs suggest that their blood sugars are averaging 154 mg/dl {9.4} throughout the entire day. If this is the average, they are likely to be experiencing post-meal blood sugar spikes that reach into the 200s.

Blood sugars that high are indeed likely to shorten your lifespan, since we know from medical research that blood sugars that spend more than a few hours each day over 140 mg/dl {7.7} will damage your heart, your nerves, your kidneys, your retinas, and your surviving beta cells.

But the outcomes for those of us who keep our blood sugars below that toxic level should be quite different. Unfortunately, no medical researcher has ever studied us. There isn't a single long term study of what happens to people with Type 2 Diabetes diagnoses who have kept their A1Cs in the 5.0-%5.9% range that correlates to average long-term blood sugars below 123 mg/dl {6.8}.

There are several reasons why this is true. One of the biggest is that so much diabetes research is funded by drug companies whose drugs don't let people achieve that kind of blood sugar control. Another reason is the extent to which diabetes care has been dominated by the belief that eating high fat diets would kill people with diabetes. The only way most of us can safely achieve those healthy 5% A1Cs is to cut back on carbs and replace some of the lost calories with fat. But academic researchers have always shied away from doing studies that would require them to feed fat to people with diabetes. That strategy is too controversial to advance an academic career.

There is one last reason why there are no studies of us people who have kept our blood sugars normal for a decade or more. Most doctors don't believe we exist—even when they see us in their practices. When we show up year after year with A1Cs in the 5% range, they assume we must have been misdiagnosed and that we never really had diabetes to start with.

Feedback I get from readers confirms me in this belief. When patients make dramatic changes in their blood sugar they may be told that their diabetes diagnoses must have been a mistake. If the diagnosis was made at an undeniably high blood sugar level, they may be told that they are some kind of freakish outlier. Rarely, if ever, do doctors ask their patients how they managed to lower their blood sugars so dramatically or how they keep them low. The self-fulfilling prophesy that people with diabetes must deteriorate keeps doctors from believing what is right before their eyes.

But quite a few of us who joined the "5% Club" 15 years ago or earlier are still here. By now some of us are in our 70s and 80s. So dismiss your fears of an early death due to your Type 2 Diabetes. Keep your blood sugar below toxic levels and you should have the same life expectancy as everyone else.

I can't guarantee you will live to be 118, or even 60. Normal people die tragically young, too. But if you get your blood sugar in line, it's possible you might live longer than many seemingly normal people whose blood sugars are rising high enough after their meals to give them heart disease.

There's one last factor working in your favor, too. People who get serious about controlling their blood sugar start eating higher quality food, become more active, and learn more about other unhealthy exposures that people with normal blood sugars are blissfully unaware of. Over time this can lead them to living a much healthier lifestyle that will also maximize their lifespan.

Will I Get Complications If My Fasting Blood Sugar isn't Normal?

On the main Blood Sugar 101 website, I posted some research that reported that when people's fasting blood sugar rises over 92 mg/dl {5.1} it becomes much more likely that they will develop diabetes over the next decade. This suggested to the researchers that 92 mg/dl is where normal fasting blood sugar ends. Another study I posted explains that our beta cells begin to experience damage when our fasting blood sugars rise over 110 mg/dl {6.1}.

Not surprisingly, I've heard from several people with diabetes who have found this information very disturbing because they can't bring their own blood sugars down that low. But if that is your situation, you needn't worry unless your *post-meal* blood sugars are also rising to levels much higher than normal.

That's because other studies suggest that the link between those slightly elevated fasting blood sugars and damage to our beta cells doesn't occur because, on their own, blood sugars over 92 or 110 mg/dl {5.1 or 6.1} are toxic. The connection is there because most people who are heading for a diabetes diagnosis only end up with fasting blood sugars that high when their *post-meal* blood sugars have already risen into the diabetic range.

When post-meal blood sugar concentrations are that high, it takes all the insulin their failing beta cells can produce to bring them back down. This makes it harder for the pancreas to make the insulin needed to cover the fasting state so that fasting blood sugar starts to rise. But it's the high post-meal blood sugars that damage the pancreas and other organs, not the much lower fasting blood sugars that go along with those post-meal highs.

As long as your fasting blood sugar is not spending a lot of time over 140 mg/dl {7.8} you should be fine. And you can lower your fasting blood sugar quite a lot by keeping your post-meal blood sugars under control. For reasons discussed on Page 123 many people with Type 2 Diabetes won't be able to get their fasting blood sugar down to completely normal levels. I certainly can't. For the past 19 years my fasting blood sugar has almost always come in around 108 mg/dl {8.0}. But I have been much more successful at controlling my post-meal blood sugars. So even 19 years into my diabetes journey my retinas, kidneys, and nerves are all doing fine. So are those of a lot of other people who struggle to lower their fasting blood sugars but are doing very well at keeping their blood sugars in the safe zone after meals.

Scientists Cured Diabetes in Mice When Will We Get This Cure?

Since I was diagnosed back in 1998 thousands of mice have been cured of diabetes. None of these cures has yet resulted in a cure for a single human with Type 2 Diabetes. To understand why, you need to know a bit about rodent research.

Mice are cheap. Mice live very short lives. So it is possible to breed many generations of mice within a few years and get them to display just about any genetic profile you choose. Mice also are expendable. Few scientists stay up late agonizing over the deaths of the mice they use in their research. These factors make them preferable to humans for research that requires feeding the subject an unapproved drug or toxic diet and then cutting the animal open to see what the drug or diet did. Hence most diabetes research is done in mice, rather than humans.

There is a problem here that scientists only discovered very recently. Rodent pancreases as well as their digestive systems are actually quite different at a molecular, genetic level from those of humans. Their enzymes are different and genes that control insulin secretion are different. This shouldn't be surprising. Mice eat very different diets in the wild than humans.

So that explains why so much of the mouse research turns out to be useless. And then there is the other, bigger problem we mentioned earlier when discussing why scientists believe that Type 2 Diabetes is caused by eating fat. Most rodent research is done with specially bred strains of mice that are described as "models" for the disease under study. Forgetful mice, who can't remember how to run a maze become models for Alzheimer's Disease, mice that get very fat on normal mouse chow become models for obesity, and sadly, mice that become diabetic when they eat "high fat diets" become models of Type 2 Diabetes. This also explains why so many of the treatments that cure these mice are useless for the 99% of people with Type 2 Diabetes whose blood sugars rise when they eat carbs, not fat.

Given what poor models mice are of human Type 2 Diabetes it should come as no surprise that almost all the drugs or other interventions that appear to cure diabetes in mice are of no use at all to humans. Our diabetes is caused by entirely different genes, responds differently to every constituent of diet, and is really a completely different condition than what is causing very high blood sugars in these rodents.

But even though these facts have emerged over the last decade, it hasn't kept scientists from continuing to do this largely irrelevant research. Professors whose entire careers have been built on mouse research continue to train new generations of mouse researchers and to make sure that the organizations funding diabetes research waste a lot of their money funding studies of these little furry "models" of diabetes.

To keep their grant money flowing, they deluge the press with press releases touting their latest cures. The press, in turn, publishes these press releases exactly as they are received, juicing up the headlines to make you click on them.

Hence, you will often see articles with headlines like "Mothers who eat meat give birth to deformed children" only to discover that it is *mouse* mothers consuming meat—which mice almost never eat and are not equipped to digest—that suffer this horrifying outcome.

Another common headline starts out "High fat diets cause..." and finishes up with something like cancer, botulism, or bad behavior in school. These, too, are mouse studies where when you look into the details of the diet that was fed to these mice, you discover that their "high fat" diet was actually a diet of corn oil mixed with a lot of high fructose corn syrup. It never seems to occur to the researchers that the corn syrup they are feeding these mice might have something to do with their unhealthy outcomes.

Very rarely, you will read about a well designed mouse study that seems to have discovered something interesting that might be applicable to humans, but you have to read the actual study very closely to determine if this is the case. Mostly, though, you should ignore any mouse research about diabetes unless you are worried about the health of a little furry pet.

Chapter Two
Why Did I Get Diabetes?

What Is Insulin Resistance?

Your doctor has undoubtedly told you that Type 2 Diabetes is characterized by high insulin resistance. But what does that term really mean?

As you probably know, insulin is the hormone that stimulates many kinds of cells, particularly muscle, fat, and liver cells, to take in glucose from your bloodstream. Once inside the cell, that glucose can be burned for energy or stored for later use in the form of fat.

The term insulin resistance describes the situation where your cells are not responding normally to insulin's signal, so it takes a much larger amount of insulin to get your cells to take in that glucose. How much larger varies from person to person, but it is very true that people with Type 2 Diabetes do need a lot more insulin to lower their blood sugar than do people, like those with Type 1 Diabetes, who are insulin sensitive.

For example, when people diagnosed with Type 2 Diabetes are put on insulin they usually need to take a dose that is between five to twenty times as much insulin as an insulin sensitive person with Type 1 Diabetes would need. This is true even when they weigh the same amount as the insulin sensitive person.

Insulin resistance has two nasty side effects. One is that the more resistant you are to insulin, the more likely you are to start experiencing high blood sugars even when you are still making near normal amounts of insulin. If you need five times more insulin than a healthy pancreas can make just to keep your blood sugar normal, your blood sugars are going to soar even when your pancreas is still making a normal amount of insulin.

The other nasty effect of insulin resistance is that fat cells keep responding to insulin's signal long after muscle cells have become insulin resistant. This is nasty because when insulin resistant fat cells take in glucose, they convert most of it into body fat. That's why insulin resistant people who eat the large amounts of carbohydrate nutritionists consider normal pack on weight so easily. It's also why many insulin resistant people find that very low carbohydrate diets are the only diets on which they can lose weight easily. When they eat these very low carb diets, most of their cells switch from burning glucose to burning fat for energy, and cells don't require insulin to burn fat.

So how do you know how insulin resistant you are? The usual way doctors measure insulin resistance is to estimate it based on the results of testing your fasting blood glucose and fasting insulin at the same time. This is done by applying a formula, called, HOMA. Medical research and my own personal experience have shown that the estimate you get from applying this formula can be completely wrong.

In my own case, the test told me I was moderately insulin resistant, but when I started using meal-time insulin I found that it took only 2 units of insulin to drop my blood sugar from 275 mg/dl {15.3} down to normal. Had I been insulin resistant, it could have taken 15 or more.

So really the only way to know how insulin resistant you are is to inject insulin and see how the amount you need compares to what other people use to achieve the same effect. For example, a person who is insulin sensitive might need no more than 12 units a day of a basal insulin to lower a high fasting blood sugar. Someone who is insulin resistant would need far more than that to lower that exact same fasting blood sugar. Typically people with Type 2 use somewhere between 25 to 300 units of basal insulin, with most people's doses clustering abound 100 units a day.

Does Insulin Resistance Cause Type 2 Diabetes?

Most doctors will tell you insulin resistance is the cause of Type 2 Diabetes. They will explain that while people with insulin-dependent Type 1 Diabetes, don't make any insulin, your body is making plenty of insulin but your cells can't use that insulin because of that insulin resistance. If you ask why you are insulin resistant you are often told it's because you are fat and that you could get rid of your Type 2 Diabetes by dieting away those extra pounds and exercising.

This is a gross overgeneralization. Though it is true that the majority of people diagnosed with Type 2 Diabetes are insulin resistant, most people who are insulin resistant *never* develop diabetes. National health surveys have found that one out of *three* Americans is insulin resistant, but only one in *ten* goes on to develop diabetes.

That's because most people with insulin resistance have normal, healthy beta cells. As their need for more insulin rises, their beta cell mass grows larger, so they are able to produce the extra insulin their insulin resistance makes necessary.

The story is quite different for insulin resistant people who go on to develop Type 2 Diabetes. Many of them turn out to have beta cells that aren't capable of functioning at full capacity. Their beta cells also fail to reproduce in response to their need for more insulin. Most importantly, both these issues appear to be due to inborn genetic problems.

So the key thing happening here is this: People who go on to develop Type 2 Diabetes have been making marginal amounts of insulin all their lives. Then when some additional stress arises that creates a demand for even more insulin, the dysfunction of their insulin-producing cells is unmasked.

The idea that obesity is the primary cause of both insulin resistance and Type 2 Diabetes is also a gross misrepresentation of what medical research has learned about Type 2 Diabetes. Two out of three Americans are overweight or obese yet, as noted above, only one in ten will ever be diagnosed with Type 2 Diabetes. This figure has remained relatively constant over the last few decades despite a huge increase in the number of Americans who have become overweight and obese.

Researchers often argue that it is fat collecting in the livers and pancreases of overweight people with diabetes that makes them insulin resistant. But this conclusion is contradicted by the discovery that slim young men whose relatives have Type 2 Diabetes turn out to be more insulin resistant than people their same size who don't have relatives with Type 2. Since these people aren't fat, fatty organs can't be blamed for their insulin resistance.

In a similar vein, I have known quite a few people with Type 2 Diabetes who have been able to get their weight down to totally normal levels who report that their insulin resistance hasn't changed as a result of that weight loss. Their insulin resistance is almost certainly genetic in origin.

And that word "genetic" is the key. Because Type 2 Diabetes turns out to be almost always the result of having inherited a collection of genes which work together to impair your ability to regulate your blood sugar. Not only that, but the more of these defective diabetic genes you have, the more likely you are to develop Type 2 diabetes.

So what do these slightly impaired diabetes-inducing genes do? A few of them—surprisingly few—do cause insulin resistance. They do this by limiting the ability of a cell to burn glucose. These cells take in a small amount of glucose when insulin levels rise, but when that glucose doesn't get burned, it piles up inside the cells. Eventually the cells put up a "Sorry Closed Until Further Notice" sign and refuse to respond to any more insulin, while they slowly and ineffectively burn through the glucose piled up inside. That's a very oversimplified version of what actually happens, but it gives you some idea of why a cell might stop responding to insulin and get you labeled "insulin resistant."

But to the surprise of researchers who had bought into the idea that it is insulin resistance that causes Type 2 Diabetes, most of the genes associated with Type 2 Diabetes have turned out to have nothing to do with insulin resistance. Instead, what they do is limit your ability to secrete insulin. There are hundreds of genetic flaws that can do this, each one affecting a different phase in the very complicated process that turns your thought, "Mmmm. smells like chocolate cake," into a squirt of insulin just the right size to take care of the glucose produced when that cake is digested.

People with a combination of genes causing both insulin resistance and insulin deficiency are likely to become fully diabetic when a new physiological stress ups the demand for insulin to a point where their marginal beta cells can't keep up. Obesity is just that kind of stress. So is pregnancy, which is why women with normal blood sugars may develop gestational diabetes, which seems to go away after their baby is born but comes back as full-fledged diabetes when they are older. So while it is true that obesity unmasks defective diabetes genes when it raises the demand for extra insulin a marginal pancreas can't supply, it doesn't actually cause it.

This strong genetic component is why Type 2 Diabetes runs in families and why if one twin develops Type 2 the other is very likely to do so, too.

Can I Lower My Insulin Resistance?

The answer here is no and yes. You're stuck with the genetic insulin resistance we just discussed. It's coded into your genes. Research suggests that you've had this kind of insulin resistance since you were born and were using more insulin than normal to process glucose even when you were a skinny little kid. The good news is that this inborn insulin resistance won't harm your body as long as you don't fill your bloodstream with more glucose than your poor, hardworking pancreas can handle.

But besides this inherited insulin resistance, there are a couple other things that can increase how much insulin resistance you have. The most important of these is the extra insulin resistance that kicks in when your blood sugar has been elevated for a while. It's a protective response your cells mount to keep from being flooded by the glucose they are being bathed in.

This acquired insulin resistance can make it much, much harder to lower your blood sugar. It becomes evident when your blood sugars reach a level somewhere between 180 and 200 mg/dl {10 and 11.1}. When your blood sugar reaches that level, it will take much more insulin to drop your blood sugar a set amount than it did when your blood sugars were lower. For example, it takes more insulin to lower your blood sugar from 250 to 220 mg/dl {13.9 to 12.8} than it would to drop it from 180 to 150 mg/dl, even though the size of the decline is the same in each case.

The good news is that this acquired insulin resistance disappears as soon as you stop loading up your blood with glucose. Once you lower your blood sugar below the threshold where acquired insulin resistance kicks in, you should see a sharp drop in your blood sugar. If you use insulin at meals, once this acquired insulin resistance clears up, you will need a lot less insulin per gram of carbohydrate you eat than you did when this additional insulin resistance was active.

If your thyroid or adrenal glands are faulty, you can also develop additional insulin resistance. There are some other medical conditions that can do this too, some quite obscure. Treating these conditions might improve this kind of acquired insulin resistance.

Insulin resistance can also increase after exposure to certain pharmaceutical drugs, including corticosteroids, SSRI antidepressants, and statins. How these substances cause insulin resistance is not well understood, nor is it known how permanent the insulin resistance is that these drugs cause. Drugs like the corticosteroids and statins appear to cause insulin resistance by limiting the function of mitochondria in our cells. Some people find that taking Co-enzyme Q10 helps combat this kind of insulin resistance. Co-enzyme Q10 helps catalyze important chemical reactions in these mitochondria.

Corticosteroid-induced insulin resistance usually goes away if you stop taking the drug, but this is not always true. It isn't clear whether the damage from statins is reversible. Once diagnosed with diabetes or metabolic syndrome people are usually put on statins, not taken off them. It isn't known why the SSRI antidepressants raise insulin resistance and raise the risk of developing diabetes. It also isn't clear whether the insulin resistance they cause can be reversed by stopping them. Some other psychiatric drugs, the atypical antipsychotics, most notably Zyprexa, cause permanent diabetes in people who had normal blood sugars before starting the drug.

The final and perhaps most potent cause of acquired insulin resistance appears to be the many industrially produced organic molecules that now pollute our food, air, and water. In many cases, the damage these chemicals do seems to be permanent because they appear to cause insulin resistance by altering genes. The most notorious example of this is the plastic BPA, which was used for baby bottles and linings of most metal food cans until very recently. Unfortunately, the chemical used to replace BPA, called BPS, appears to be equally harmful. Animal studies have found that the insulin resistance caused by exposure to BPA gets passed down not only to offspring of exposed mothers, but to those offspring's' offspring. This causes obesity in all three generations studied. It's quite possible that the high concentration of plastic-related chemicals like BPA in our food and water go a long way towards explaining the obesity epidemic and why it is affecting so many young children.

Other environmental toxins that cause both insulin resistance and increased rates of diabetes in those exposed to them include PCBs, the plasticizers found in items like shampoo bottles, flame retardants, anti-stick compounds, and a long list of herbicides and pesticides. If these chemicals are causing insulin resistance by damaging genes, it won't be reversible. If it is only causing it by stimulating receptors, which may be the case with some, it may be.

Why Does Dr. _____ Claim He Can Lower Insulin Resistance?

As you learned earlier, you can eliminate the acquired insulin resistance caused by running a higher than normal blood sugar — one over 180 mg/dl {10}, but you are stuck with insulin resistance caused by your genes.

Diets that lower blood sugar — which are usually diets with limited amounts of carbohydrate — will get rid of the acquired form of insulin resistance, but that is all they can do. I am not aware of any published study that has conclusively shown that a diet resulted in a *permanent* reduction in cellular insulin resistance, once the dieter went off the carb-restricted diet that lowered their blood sugars below the point where that acquired insulin resistance kicks in.

Sometimes researchers will base a claim that their diet reduced insulin resistance based on the estimates of insulin resistance they get from applying the HOMA formula to measures of fasting blood sugar and fasting glucose. However, both fasting blood sugar and fasting insulin will drop after a person lowers their carbs significantly, which is what most of these diets make people do. Both will almost always rise back to their original levels if people go back to eating the high carb diet normal people can handle. My guess is that the HOMA formula is only predictive of insulin resistance when people are eating that standard diet with its 300 grams of carbohydrate a day.

Some proponents of weight loss surgery claim that their surgery cures Type 2 Diabetes and lowers insulin resistance. But this intervention also appears to be effective only as long as it reduces the amount of carbohydrate a person can fit into their digestive tract. When you can't eat carbs, your blood sugar will drop like a stone. But this "cure" vanishes for most people, no matter how much weight they have lost, as soon as their stomach stretches out enough to allow them to boost their carb intake.

When I polled people with Type 2 Diabetes who had lost a lot of weight, asking them if their ability to tolerate carbohydrates had increased a very few said yes. The rest reported that if they raised their carbs their blood sugars went back to their previous levels. This suggests that their innate insulin resistance had not changed.

Does Eating Fat Cause Type 2 Diabetes?

Rodent research has convinced a lot of doctors and nutritionists that people get Type 2 Diabetes because they eat too much fat. But a closer look at that research makes it clear that what it *really* proves is that *genetically modified rodents* get diabetes when they eat too much fat. And we aren't talking just any old mutant rodent here. The rodents that star in diabetes research are mutant rodents that were chosen to be models for human Type 2 Diabetes precisely because these rodents get diabetes when they eat fat.

So what we have here is some brilliantly circular reasoning. Rodents selected to be a model for human Type 2 Diabetes *because* they get diabetes when they eat fat are fed fat and get diabetes—which is used to "prove" that humans get diabetes because they eat fat.

In fact, the genes that make these particular mutant rodents get diabetes are not the genes found in humans who get Type 2 Diabetes— who, it turns out, mostly get diabetes when they eat too much *carbohydrate*, not fat.

But it's likely that carbs they ate also played a bigger role than the researchers realized in the sorry fate of those poor little diabetic rodents. Because it also turns out that the "high fat diet" that these rodents are fed is not only high in fat but is also rich in carbohydrates since it's full of corn syrup. So rather than eating a "high fat diet," which is what you see in the headlines, these rodents were eating a high carb/high fat diet, one providing enough carbs to cause all the problems attributed to the diet's high fat content.

Bad science like this couldn't have passed scrutiny had it not been for the religiously held belief of everyone in the medical community that it was the fat we eat that was to blame for all our ills. It was an easy mistake to make. People in ill health do have a lot of fat where it doesn't belong: surrounding their organs, clogging their arteries, and inflaming their livers. High levels of fat in the blood—the triglycerides that show up on their cholesterol test results—can be predictive of heart disease.

But what these fat-phobic researchers failed to account for was this: most of the damaging fat that circulates in our blood and ends up infiltrating our organs doesn't come from the fat we eat. It comes from eating too many *carbs*.

That's because once your liver has stored up enough glucose to get you through a few days without food it converts any unneeded starches or sugars you eat to triglycerides—those damaging blood fats. Cut down on the carbs and those blood triglycerides plunge. People eating almost no carbs can consume a diet that is 68% fat and still get perfect triglyceride values on their cholesterol tests. I've done it and I know quite a few other people who have done the same thing. Some larger men can eat a diet that is as much as 80% fat with 10% carbs and have normal blood triglycerides.

This little understood explanation of what raises blood fats explains why decades of research were never able to show that a low fat diet prevented heart disease. How could it? The low fat diet was of necessity very high in carbs and those excess carbs got converted to the damaging triglycerides that accumulated in the arteries and caused heart disease.

Recent research has even found some hints that consumption of dairy fat—the saturated stuff you find in butter, cream, and cheese—seems to be correlated with a lower risk of getting diabetes. Could that be because it is a marker for diets lower in carb and higher in fat that don't stress our pancreases so much?

If you want to see some of the large body of research that has called into question the demonization of fat read this page on my main website: "Studies Proving the Safety and Efficacy of Low Carb Diets." You'll find it at **http://www.bloodsugar101.com/19066498.php**.

Does Prediabetes Always Turn into Diabetes?

Told that they have prediabetes many people wonder if this means they are doomed to develop Type 2 Diabetes. Most won't. Insulin resistance can lead to blood sugars rising into the prediabetic range. But as we mentioned earlier, though the US National Institutes of Health tell us that almost one in three Americans have prediabetes, fewer than one in ten people will ever develop full-fledged diabetes, despite what you hear about the so-called "diabetes epidemic."

As we also mentioned earlier, the people who go on to develop full-fledged diabetes after getting a prediabetes diagnosis are almost always those who have some additional problem that limits ability of their beta cells to secrete insulin and reproduce. Usually these problems are caused by inherited genetic problems. Occasionally they are caused by toxic exposures to chemicals that damage the beta cells.

But even if you are one of the lucky people whose prediabetes never advances to something more serious, you should not be too complacent, because even if you never have to worry about the classic diabetic complications, you do have to worry about heart disease. And as you'll recall, heart disease starts becoming more common when people's blood sugars are only rising into the prediabetic blood sugar range. There is some evidence that most of the heart disease supposedly normal people get is caused by undiagnosed prediabetes.

Why Did My Fasting Blood Sugar Suddenly Hit 300?

A surprising number of us get our diabetes diagnoses after having been given no previous warning. One day our family doctor runs a routine blood test and the next thing we know we are given that shocking diagnosis.

Does diabetes really develop that quickly? For a few of us—those of us who have come down with autoimmune diabetes—the answer is yes. The autoimmune attack that destroys your pancreas can happen very quickly. But Type 2 Diabetes develops much more slowly. We just don't know it because the warnings that should have alerted us get missed. That's because early Type 2 Diabetes is invisible to the tests doctors use to screen for diabetes.

Many of us develop diabetes in a pattern where our blood sugars rise very steeply after we eat long before our fasting blood sugar reaches a level that would catch a doctor's attention. Because our fasting blood sugar remains just barely above normal, our A1C stays in the prediabetic range, too—somewhere between 5.7 and 6.4%.

No test doctors use for screening ever looks at how high our blood sugar is rising after we eat. So those post-meal highs may go on for years before they rise high enough to be detected. All the while, though, they are damaging our blood vessels and killing off our beta cells. Eventually enough cells have died that our fasting blood sugar rises high enough that our doctor will give us a diagnosis.

A less common pattern in which diabetes develops is one where fasting blood sugars deteriorate before post-meal readings. But you may get little warning here, either, since fasting blood sugar doesn't worsen in a gradual or linear fashion. It may stay prediabetic for ever, which is why many doctors will ignore a prediabetic fasting blood sugar, or it may stay prediabetic for years and then, over two or three years, shoot up dramatically.

Even when we register a solidly prediabetic test value, some doctors still may not mention it to us. I hear from quite a few people who have had this happen. This may occur because a lot of people with prediabetes never go on to develop diabetes, so doctors figure that since there is nothing they can prescribe to treat prediabetes there's no real point in wasting valuable time by bringing it up. They know from experience that telling patients to eat a healthier diet will be futile—that low fat diet full of oatmeal and bananas—since almost none of their patients can ever lose weight.

Then, too, the ADA guidelines have taught doctors that A1Cs below 7.0% are nothing to worry about. So when your screening test comes through with a prediabetic value, they may just make a note on your chart to keep an eye on it at your next annual checkup, but don't mention the test result to you. That way they can use the limited time they have to spend with you discussing something they consider more important—like a high cholesterol test.

One final reason you may get no warning until your blood sugar has risen to alarming heights is that older family doctors who received their training before 1998 were taught that the fasting blood sugar level at which they should diagnose diabetes was 140 mg/dl {7.8}. From what people have reported to me, some still wait until your fasting blood sugar has risen that high before telling you that you're diabetic and urging you to take action.

Even when they do give you a diagnosis, some older, out-of-touch doctors may treat what they call "mild diabetes" as if it weren't important. Not that long ago, a beloved small town doctor diagnosed someone I know and then just told him, "Don't eat white foods." I had to wonder how many of his patients had dutifully switched from vanilla to chocolate ice cream.

Does Reactive Hypoglycemia Lead to Type 2 Diabetes?

Some of us have gotten an early warning sign that we were on the road to developing Type 2 Diabetes, but our doctors brushed it off as unimportant. That warning sign was that we started experiencing low blood sugar attacks a few hours after eating.

The medical term for this is "reactive hypoglycemia." These attacks can make you feel shaky and nervous and their effects can linger for a few hours, even if you raise your blood sugar by eating something sugary. Though you might feel the symptoms of reactive hypoglycemia at normal blood sugar levels, you aren't considered officially hypoglycemic unless your blood sugar test value is below 70 mg/dl {3.9}.

Reactive hyperglycemia is often the very first hint a person gets that their blood sugar is no longer entirely normal. It can happen a decade or more before the person is diagnosed with diabetes. To understand why reactive hypoglycemia is a hint that your blood sugar control is eroding you need to understand how normal healthy blood sugar control works.

When a totally normal person eats a meal full of carbs, their pancreas secretes a burst of insulin as soon as they start thinking about eating. Then about an hour after their meal, if their blood sugar hasn't gone back to its usual fasting level, their pancreas starts a second, slower, more prolonged bout of insulin secretion that continues until any excess glucose has been removed from the blood.

But what happens when your blood sugar control is just beginning to slip, is that the early burst of insulin that is supposed to happen at the beginning of the meal starts weakening. So the carbs in your meal push your blood sugar up to a level slightly higher than normal level. As your blood sugar rises over its normal post-meal high,, your pancreas responds by releasing a stronger than usual second burst of insulin which not only takes care of the high but overshoots its target, sending you low.

Not every one who gets hypoglycemic attacks goes on to develop Type 2 Diabetes. Some may have normal insulin production and their hypos result from some other cause. But in the many people who do experience these hypos, what happens after a year or so of hypoglycemic attacks is this: their hypoglycemia goes away. The hypos stop, the person feels better, and completely forgets about their blood sugar.

But the hypos have stopped only because their pancreas is no longer able to make the extra large bursts of insulin that were dropping their blood sugar into the hypo range. So their blood sugar is still spiking high after meals, because they are making less and less of that early burst of insulin normal people secrete.

As their blood sugars rise higher after meals, the person may start having trouble controlling their appetite, as blood sugars shooting up and dropping steeply make many of us hungry. But it may take another decade until their blood sugars reach a level high that the ADA guidelines would flag them as prediabetic.

Fortunately, if you think you have reactive hypoglycemia, or if you had it in the past and it has disappeared, you don't need a doctor's help to determine if your blood sugar is rising high after meals. Just buy yourself an inexpensive blood sugar meter—how to do that is discussed in the next chapter.

Test your blood sugar one hour after you eat one of the meals that was giving you the reactive hypos. If you see several readings over 160 mg/dl {8.9}, it is likely that your ability to secrete insulin is beginning to weaken. The good news is that you have discovered this very early, at a time when you still have lots of insulin secreting capability left.

It's very easy to correct this problem at this early stage. Just follow the "Test, Test, Test" strategy described in the next chapter, but when you do it, try to get down to totally normal blood sugars after meals, rather than the slightly higher blood sugars that are suggested for people diagnosed with diabetes who may be able to attain lower ones.

If you do discuss reactive hypoglycemia with a doctor, they are likely to tell you to eat more protein, which is not helpful advice when you are in the middle of a hypoglycemic attack. When your blood sugar is low what you need to boost it is carbs. Protein won't do anything to head off a developing hypo.

But you only need a very small amount of carbohydrate to correct a hypo. If you do what most people do and chug a big glass of orange juice or soda, or eat a handful of cookies, you are likely to cause a second blood sugar spike that will cause another reactive hypo. The best way to correct a hypo is to take just enough glucose to raise your blood sugar 20 or 30 mg/dl {1.1 or 1.7}. This should put it back to the middle of the normal fasting range. You can read about how to do that in the discussion of mild hypoglycemia you'll find on Page 114.

To prevent hypos watch your carbs. Eating less carb and more fat will keep hypos from happening. The advice doctors give recommending that you eat more protein is yet another result of the fat phobia that has perverted nutritional advice for so long. Doctors couldn't just come out and tell people to cut their carbs, because then they might eat more of that deadly fat. So instead they told them to eat protein.

We know now that if you cut your carbs down to a level that gives you completely normal blood sugars, there is nothing wrong with eating a mix of protein and healthy fats. Just go easy on the carbs.

Does My Gestational Diabetes Mean I'll Get Type 2?

Pregnancy puts a huge strain on your metabolism, so if your pancreas is just barely keeping up with your insulin needs before you get pregnant, the additional demands of pregnancy can be far more than it can handle. This leads to a diagnosis of gestational diabetes.

Doctors describe gestational diabetes as if it were a different condition from regular diabetes, one that goes away after the baby is born. But research has found that women with gestational diabetes almost always have the same genes as women who develop Type 2 Diabetes later in life. There are a few exceptions to this. A very small group of women who develop gestational diabetes turn out to be in the very early stages of a slow, adult-onset form of autoimmune diabetes—a form of Type 1—that is becoming more frequent among adults. An even tinier group experience gestational diabetes because they were born with one of a number of rare genetic forms of diabetes that has given them prediabetic blood sugars all their lives. Their blood sugars then become diabetic under the stress of pregnancy.

In an ideal world, doctors would urge women who have had diabetic pregnancies to work as hard on controlling their blood sugar after their baby is born as they did when it was in the womb. They'd give them prescriptions for meters and strips and urge them to cut back on their carbs to protect their already struggling insulin secreting cells. But this rarely happens.

Though OB/GYNs are refreshingly aware of the importance of tight blood sugar control, women go back to their family doctors once their baby is delivered. Those doctors ignore their blood sugars as long as their screening tests don't turn up fasting blood glucose readings high enough for a diabetes diagnosis.

But if *you* have been diagnosed with gestational diabetes, you should not ignore it. Instead, treat it as a lucky break. You have been given a very early warning that your pancreas is stressed and can barely keep up with the demands you have been putting on it. If you heed this warning and make some simple changes to your diet, you may be able to protect your remaining insulin secreting cells and keep from ever developing Type 2 Diabetes. If you ignore this warning and wait until your blood sugar has gotten bad enough to show up on your annual screening tests it will be a lot harder to bring your blood sugars back down to normal. So be proactive after a diagnosis of gestational diabetes.

Here is the checklist I tell women to follow when they ask me what to do after a diagnosis of gestational diabetes:

❖ Once your baby is born, cut back on the carbs! This can be tough to do when you have infants and toddlers to deal with, but it is well worth doing. The fewer demands you make on your beta cells now the better your blood sugar will be when your baby heads off to high school.

❖ Once or twice a year, get out your meter and test your blood sugar one hour and two hours after you eat a bagel, potato, or portion of rice that contains about 70 grams of carbohydrate. This stress test is similar to a glucose tolerance test. It should give you a good idea of whether your blood sugar control is remaining normal or slowly progressing towards diabetes.

❖ If you see readings over 200 mg/dl {11.1} at any time when you test your blood sugar at home, assume that you are diabetic no matter what your doctor might say. The official document instructing doctors how to diagnose people with diabetes states explicitly that several readings over that level, recorded at any time of the day, should lead to a diagnosis of Type 2 Diabetes. Then use the technique you'll find described in the next chapter to get your blood sugars back down into the normal range.

I Have Always Eaten a Healthy Diet Why Did I Get Diabetes?

One of the first things you will learn after you get yourself a blood sugar meter and start testing your blood sugar after eating is that diet you have been told is a "healthy diet" raises your blood sugars to extremely unhealthy heights.

The typical diet most nutritionists recommend is full of starchy grains, beans, and root vegetables and sugary fruits. It isn't unusual for a single "healthy" meal to contain 100 grams of carbohydrate. How unhealthy this really is comes into focus when you learn that 100 grams is two or three times as much carbohydrate as most people with *prediabetic* blood sugar can eat without seeing a significant post-meal blood sugar spike.

Testing your blood sugar is likely to reveal that a diet full of delicious unprocessed cheeses and juicy steaks is a lot healthier for us than the skim milk, quinoa, beets, and sugary salad dressings we've been snookered into thinking are health food. So let's redefine healthy:

The only healthy diet for a person with diabetes is one that doesn't raise their blood sugar.

I'm Thin—Why Was I Diagnosed with Type 2?

There are several reasons why a person of normal weight might be diagnosed with Type 2 Diabetes. One is that they are not descended from people who spent many generations living in Western Europe. Most of the research on Type 2 Diabetes has been done only in people with that background, so doctors assume that what has been learned about Type 2 Diabetes as it appears in that population applies to everyone who gets it.

But it turns out that the genes that cause diabetes in people from different ethnic backgrounds are different for each ethnic group. The way their diabetes develops and the way it affects their bodies can be quite different from the Western European norm. For example, people from Japan are likely to develop diabetes without the dramatic obesity often seen in people of Western European heritage.

The genes that govern diabetes in Western European Jewish populations also seem to differ from those of other Western European populations. This population can develop Type 2 Diabetes at lower body weights than some other Western European groups.

The other major reason why people of normal weight might be diagnosed with Type 2 Diabetes is that they have been misdiagnosed. There are two different completely unrelated forms of diabetes that are often misdiagnosed as Type 1.

The first is a slow-developing form of autoimmune diabetes that is very similar to Type 1 Diabetes but has a few genetic characteristics that make it more like Type 2. This is called Latent Autoimmune Diabetes of Adults, usually abbreviated as LADA. People with LADA are usually, but not always, insulin sensitive. Though at diagnosis many people with LADA can get by without using insulin, within five years most will require it, as the slow autoimmune attack on their pancreas destroys their ability to make insulin. Very tight control won't stop this progression, nor does it help to start insulin immediately after diagnosis when there is still a significant population of living beta cells.

The incidence of LADA seems to have increased dramatically over the past 20 years. There is probably an environmental reason for this. Some believe it is because we are spending the childhood years when the immune system develops living in environments that are too clean. Without exposure to the bacteria and other organisms found in dirt, the immune system doesn't focus on external invaders but shifts into a mode where it is more likely to turn on our own tissues.

Another possible explanation for the surge in LADA may be additives to our food that damage our gut linings and allow large proteins like those found in milk to enter the bloodstream. The similarities these large protein molecules share with our beta cells may provoke the immune system to attack both the food proteins and the beta cells. The highly processed soy proteins added to so many processed foods appear to cause this damage to our intestines known as "leaky gut syndrome," too.

LADA tends to progress slowly at first, so it won't immediately land you in the emergency room the way Type 1 can. But if you ignore it, a few years later it *will* become an emergency. If you think you might have LADA, watch your post-meal blood sugars carefully. If they are climbing so that the same meal that used to raise your blood sugar to, say, 250 mg/dl {13.9} starts raising it to 300 mg/dl {16.7}, inform your doctor and ask for a referral to an endocrinologist who can order the tests that will determine if LADA is causing this deterioration. Even if your insurer doesn't require that you get a referral, it's best to contact an endocrinologist with a referral in hand. That referral may get you seen faster than someone who makes their own appointment. It also makes the endo take your concerns more seriously since the referral means your family doctor is also concerned.

Doctors often fail to recognize the signs of autoimmune diabetes when it strikes middle aged people who like their normal peers are likely to be overweight or obese. Doctors are very influenced by society's stereotypes, so they tend to often assume that any diabetes found in a fat person must be Type 2.

That said, not all normal weight people with diabetes who don't respond well to Type 2 drugs have LADA. Some really do have classic Type 2 Diabetes caused by the diabetic genes that limit their ability to secrete insulin. Not all are insulin resistant. Some are, but through diligent dieting have been able to keep their weight under control.

There are also some much rarer forms of diabetes that are also misdiagnosed as Type 2. These are caused by specific genetic errors, so if you have one, you would have had it all your life. Even so, some of these rare genetic forms don't get diagnosed until you are an adult, because they only cause mildly impaired blood sugars when you are young—ones too low to be detected by the screening tests doctors use.

Like regular Type 2 Diabetes these rare forms may only get diagnosed when more stress is put on your blood sugar control by factors like menopause, significant weight gain, a toxic exposure, the use of a drug that worsens insulin resistance, or normal aging. These forms of diabetes are often lumped together under the term MODY diabetes.

Could I Have MODY Diabetes?

Since I first started writing about MODY diabetes, I have often heard from people with Type 2 diagnoses whose emails make it sound like they are really hoping they have it. My suspicion is that this is because they feel that a diagnosis of an exotic form of diabetes would remove the stigma associated with having plain old, boring Type 2.

But very few people really have MODY diabetes. It is rare and if you have it, the chances are very good that you would have had hints throughout your whole life that your blood sugar wasn't normal. Women with MODY are very likely to develop gestational diabetes though they start out their pregnancies at completely normal weights. Both men and women with it will be victimized by recurring fungal infections like vaginal yeast, athlete's foot, and crotch rot. In their teens, people with MODY may have had far more cavities than normal due to the abnormally high amounts of glucose in their saliva.

People with these forms of diabetes rarely are insulin resistant and will not respond strongly to drugs that lower insulin resistance like metformin or Actos. People who have two particular versions of MODY will, however, respond very strongly to drugs that stimulate insulin production, like glipizide, glimepiride, glyburide, repaglinide, Januvia and Onglyza.

MODY can only be formally diagnosed with expensive gene tests that insurance may not cover. But if you can't get tested, a misdiagnosis is by no means a crisis. In fact, with some versions of MODY getting a correct diagnosis may make it harder, not easier, to improve your health.

Doctors have misinterpreted a research study about one of the more common forms of this uncommon condition, MODY-2, in a way that makes them now believe it requires no treatment at all. That's because people with MODY-2 rarely develop the classic diabetic complications. What they do develop, unfortunately, after a lifetime of exposure to prediabetic blood sugars, is severe heart disease that kills a lot of them in their 40s or 50s.

In the case of two other forms of MODY, doctors have decided it's better for people who have it to control the very high blood sugars characteristic of these conditions with cheap insulin-stimulating pills, which many patients find very hard to tolerate, in place of the expensive insulin shots or pumps that work a whole lot better.

So getting diagnosed with any of these forms of MODY, may lead to your doctor taking away your prescriptions for the drugs and devices that have hitherto served you very well, leaving you with no treatment at all or a treatment that leaves you hungry all the time with very unpredictable blood sugars.

The only reason to look for a MODY diagnosis is if your family has a history of early kidney disease—which is a symptom of some of these forms of genetic diabetes, or if you are having an extremely hard time controlling your blood sugar along with other usual symptoms that might point to your having one of the more obscure forms of MODY. But as long as your blood sugars are under control using the drugs your doctor prescribes because they think you have a form of

Type 2 that isn't responding to most oral drugs, there is no reason to get an official diagnosis.

You can read much more about these very rare forms of diabetes on the web page "MODY - it's Not Type 1 or Type 2 but Something Else" that you'll find at **http://www.bloodsugar101.com/14047009.php**..

Could Another Autoimmune Disease Cause Diabetes?

Thyroid problems can cause insulin resistance to rise, which can push up marginally normal blood sugars into the pre- or fully diabetic range. So it is quite possible for people with autoimmune thyroid disease to develop classic Type 2 Diabetes, the kind where they are making lots of insulin but still experiencing high blood sugars.

But people with other autoimmune diseases are also more likely to develop the autoimmune forms of diabetes which may or may not involve insulin resistance. This is because they are likely to have faulty immune system genes that make it easier to get any autoimmune disease.

Rising blood sugars in someone with an autoimmune disease don't always mean that their immune system is attacking their pancreases. Sometimes systemic inflammation caused by the original immune problem can spread to the pancreas and limit its ability to secrete insulin. So people with Multiple Sclerosis, Lupus, and Rheumatoid Arthritis may see their blood sugars rise into the diabetic range when their conditions flare up but improve later when their autoimmune condition goes into remission.

If you have been diagnosed with another autoimmune disease and are given a diagnosis of Type 2 Diabetes, ask your doctor to run the tests that distinguish between autoimmune diabetes and other forms. The fasting insulin or C-peptide tests are the most commonly ordered screening tests. There are also tests that can determine if you have developed the antibodies characteristic of autoimmune diabetes.

Because my website discusses the adult onset form of Type 1 Diabetes, I often get emails from people who sound like they are hoping they really have autoimmune diabetes (Type 1) rather than Type 2, even though their blood sugar drops dramatically when they cut their carbs. That is not what happens to people with autoimmune diabetes whose beta cells are mostly dead.

This is a measure of just how toxic the media image of Type 2 Diabetes has become. People desperately hope they don't have Type 2 because of the shame associated with that diagnosis. But the truth is, if there is any question about your diagnosis, you should fervently hope that you *do* have Type 2. Type 1 might not carry a stigma, but it is much, much tougher to manage. People with Type 1 envy those with Type 2 because, to them, their lives seem so much easier.

You can read more about the slow onset autoimmune diabetes adults get on this web page: LADA—"Slow Adult Onset Autoimmune Diabetes with Some Type 2 Features." You'll find that page at **http://www.bloodsugar101.com/18382053.php.**

What Does My C-Peptide Test Result Mean?

The C-peptide test is a very crude test. The only results that are meaningful, or even reproducible, are those that are at the very high end of your lab's reference range and those at the very low end. If you have a high fasting blood glucose test result at the same time you have an extremely low C-peptide test result, it suggests you are secreting almost no insulin. In that case, you should have further tests to see if you are developing a form of Type 1 Diabetes. C-peptide test results that come in towards the top of the lab's reference range suggest that you are making quite a bit of insulin and that insulin resistance is causing your high blood sugars. Anything in-between means only that you are still making insulin. An increase in the reported value from one C-peptide test to another doesn't mean that your blood sugar control is worsening. The same blood sample tested for C-peptide twice on the same day can yield very different results if the result falls within that intermediate range.

If your C-peptide test results are low, it doesn't necessarily mean that you have a form of Type 1 Diabetes. But it should make your doctor either order antibody tests to see if you have developed the antibodies used to diagnose autoimmune diabetes or send you to an endocrinologist who can do this.

How Can I Stop Feeling So Awful About Giving Myself this Terrible Disease?

The media have long promoted the false belief that people get Type 2 Diabetes because they are fat and lazy. No wonder a diagnosis can make you feel guilty and ashamed. How awful to have given yourself a terrible disease just because you couldn't stop being a lazy glutton.

This is utter baloney. But it is really toxic baloney, because most people deal with guilt and shame by going into a state of denial. This is toxic because when you go into denial about your diabetes, you won't take the steps you need to take to keep it from harming your body.

The best way to heal these destructive, negative emotions is to educate yourself about what actually causes Type 2 Diabetes. Earlier answers in this chapter have already sketched out the major causes of the genetic damage that leads to Type 2 Diabetes: inherited genes, acquired genetic damage, and organ damage from toxic exposures. If you want to read about all these causes and several more in greater depth, I suggest you visit this web page "You Did NOT Eat Your Way to Diabetes: The REAL Causes" at:

http://www.bloodsugar101.com/14046739.php.

Some people have written to me protesting that they know for sure that they *did* cause their diabetes because they ate like pigs before they got diagnosed. I always reply that I have no doubt that they did. Where I differ with them, though, is that I don't believe it was any personal moral weakness that led them to do to this.

Why? Because I know both from personal experience and reading research that the roller coaster blood sugars we experience in the earlier stages of the process that leads to Type 2 Diabetes can cause us to become ravenously, almost insanely hungry.

When our blood sugars surge up to 250 mg/dl {13.9} and then plummet down 150 points to a normal fasting blood sugar, we can experience extreme, uncontrollable hunger that will make us want to eat all the time. A few years of this kind of hunger will pack on the excess weight most of us are carrying when we are diagnosed.

If you eliminate those blood sugar spikes by cutting way back on the large portions of sugar and starchy foods that cause them, that hunger will go away. This usually happens very fast—within a week or two, and when your blood sugar flattens out and that obsessive hunger fades away, you will finally understand that the ravenous hunger you thought was your own personal gluttony was just your blood sugar making you crazy. Once you know that, you will stop beating yourself up or feeling like a helpless addict and do what you have to do to keep that relentless hunger from ever returning again.

My Doctor Says I *Don't* Have Type 2 Diabetes What Should I Do?

As I mentioned earlier, doctors rarely will diagnose you with diabetes until your fasting blood glucose is over 125 mg/dl {6.9} or your A1C is over 6.5%. They rarely order any tests that check out post-meal blood sugars, though it is these post-meal levels that deteriorate first in many people who eventually are diagnosed with Type 2 Diabetes.

Even when you tell your doctor that your home testing is showing repeated readings over 200 mg/dl {11.1}, your doctor may brush them off, as unimportant. You may think this means you need to find a new doctor—one who will be more supportive of your desire to improve your health. But it may be impossible to switch doctors. Your insurance plan may force you to remain under their care, as may your government health care system. Or you may not want to switch because your current doctor might be very good at treating some other health condition you have that requires more actual care from a doctor than does diabetes.

If you can't get an early diagnosis, there's no reason to fire your doctor right away, because there is very little that any doctor can do for you this early in the progress of diabetes. The only truly helpful thing a doctor could do, besides give you a prescription for blood sugar test strips, might be to give you a prescription for metformin. Metformin is a safe, very cheap generic drug which is also indicated as a treatment for prediabetes. But even without a diagnosis, if you nag, most doctors will write you those prescriptions, even if they think you are a hypochondriac. Few patients ask for test strips, so insurers haven't yet strong-armed doctors into refusing to prescribe them.

The rest of the drugs doctors are likely to prescribe for people just diagnosed with Type 2 Diabetes are pretty toxic. The most effective, safe intervention this early stage of blood sugar dysfunction is to change your diet in the way we recommend in the next chapter.

But if you feel like your doctor isn't taking you seriously, when you feel sure that you do have diabetes, it helps to know that there is a good reason why your doctor may be behaving this way. The world is full of people who are convinced, for one reason or another, that they have diabetes even though their blood sugars are in fact, completely normal.

I hear from quite a few of them. Some are desperately hoping that they have diabetes because they have some other painful condition no doctor can diagnose or treat. Their thinking is that if their symptoms are caused by diabetes, they can be cured by diabetes treatments. Others are full-fledged hypochondriacs—people with nothing really wrong with them who obsess about their health and imagine every vague symptom is an emergency. So if your doctor dismisses your reports of high blood sugars on home testing, it is possible they have had to deal with too many patients like that.

It's also worth repeating that if your fasting blood sugars are under 125 mg/dl {6.9}, your A1C is under 6.5%, and your post-meal blood sugars are always under 200 mg/dl {11.1} you really *don't* have diabetes. You might have prediabetes, but if that's the case there really isn't anything a doctor can do to help you. Cutting back on how many carbs you eat is the safest and most effective treatment for prediabetes.

Chapter Three
How Do I Lower My Blood Sugar?

What Should My Doctor Prescribe at Diagnosis?

There is one essential tool your doctor should prescribe when you are diagnosed with Type 2 Diabetes: a blood sugar meter. They will also need to prescribe as many blood sugar test strips as your insurance will permit you to have. Your blood sugar meter is the single most powerful weapon you have with which to win the battle against Type 2 Diabetes. Since the blood sugar test strips your meter uses are very expensive, it really helps to have your doctor write the prescription that will get your insurance company paying for them. If you are on Medicare, with a prescription, your meter and small supply of test strips will be free.

But many doctors don't think to offer prescriptions for testing supplies to patients diagnosed with Type 2 Diabetes, unless they are taking medications that can cause dangerous hypos. That's because doctors have been told that studies have supposedly proven that people with Type 2 Diabetes don't lower their blood sugars when they monitor their blood sugars at home with a meter. Insurers love these studies, as they give them a pretext to deny covering expensive testing supplies. That may be why so many doctors are now aware of these studies.

Mind you, these studies really did take place and the people in them who were given meters and expensive test strips really weren't able to lower their blood sugars. But there is a very simple explanation for why these people got such poor results:

The researchers in these studies told the study subjects to test their blood sugar first thing in the morning—not after meals. Perhaps they told them to test that way because they didn't understand where the instructions to test only fasting blood sugars came from. These are the instructions doctors are supposed to give to patients who are prescribed basal insulin, a kind of insulin which only lowers fasting blood sugars. Patients using these insulins do need to test their blood sugar first thing in the morning because if their fasting blood sugar is too high or too low, they will need to adjust the dose of their basal insulin to fix it.

But when a patient is *not* injecting insulin and is controlling their blood sugar entirely through diet, they have no way of lowering their *fasting* blood sugars. The only blood sugars they can lower are the ones that occur after meals.

Just observing those high post-meal blood sugars won't bring them down, of course. Patients also need to be taught that the carbs they eat are what raise those post-meal blood sugars and that the way to lower their blood sugars is to eat less carbs. With that information, patients whose blood sugar testing shows unacceptably high blood sugars can take effective action.

Weirdly, many doctors I have spoken with over the years are not aware that it's the carbs we eat and only the carbs that raise blood sugars. Nor do they know that cutting carbs will drop blood sugar better than any drug currently on the market. One endocrinologist actually told me that it was eating *fat* that raised people's blood sugars!

Perhaps doctors are unaware of the impact of carbs on blood sugar because these very healthy Type A people have blood sugars so normal that if they test themselves after a meal full of carbs they don't see any spike. Or maybe it's just because they've never tested their own blood sugar. I have heard from quite a few doctors who have been just as surprised as the rest of us to be told out of the blue that they had developed full-fledged diabetes.

Because doctors don't understand the value of the feedback you get from testing your blood sugar after eating you may have to put some pressure on your doctor to get the prescription you need for testing supplies. If you encounter resistance, ask for one month's worth and tell the doctor that if you haven't dropped your A1C by 1% at your next appointment, they can cancel the prescription. Then work your butt off to get your blood sugars down.

If you follow the strategy laid out in the next section, that 1% drop should be easy. You may very well drop it a lot more, especially if your A1C is closer to 8% than 6%. An open-minded, supportive doctor will give you that prescription. If yours won't, look for a more helpful doctor if the health coverage you have makes changing doctors a possibility.

What Is the Best Brand of Meter?

People always ask me "Which meter should I use?" But I can't tell you what's the best meter to buy because a) none of them is all that accurate, b) unless you have Cadillac insurance your choice of meters may be limited to what your insurer will pay for or what you can afford, and c) meter companies keep changing their products.

I don't test any but the cheapest and the ones my insurer will pay for. But even if I could, by the time you read this book, the one I might have recommended may have been replaced by another model.

The good news is that you don't need the "best" meter to lower your blood sugar. All you need is a meter that is consistent with itself. By consistent with itself I mean that if you test your blood sugar once and see a reading of 125 mg/dl {6.9} a second reading taken immediately from the same test site should not be more than 5 mg/dl [.3} higher or lower.

The changes in your diet that are going to make the most impact on your health are those that bring your one hour post-meal blood sugars down from readings like 300, 275, 250, 225 or 200 mg/dl to a reading near in the low to middle 100s. {16.6 to 5.5}. Do that and you will see your A1C drop into the 6% range or lower. If your not-so-good but consistent meter reads 325 mg/dl when a lab draw would have read 300 mg/dl, and your blood sugar meter later reads 160 mg/dl instead of the 135 mg/dl you'd see at a lab, you've still made the kind of change you need to make to recover your health.

If you worry that that 160 mg/dl you're seeing on your meter might actually be much higher, not lower, than your real blood glucose concentration, take your meter with you to the lab the next time your doctor orders a comprehensive metabolic panel. That's a common test doctors often order at your annual checkup. The metabolic panel includes a glucose test. Measure your blood sugar right before or after the lab draw and write down the number. Comparing your meter's reading with the lab draw will tell you whether your meter is reading high or low and give you a rough idea of by how much.

Do I Have to Do a Control Solution Test?

Meters always come with instructions telling the buyer to run control solution tests to validate that the meter is accurate. But these tests are a complete waste of strips. Meters that are reading 20, 30, or more mg/dl higher than a simultaneous lab draw always test within the proper range when you waste test strips on the control solution test that meter companies instruct you to do. I have experienced this myself and have received quite a few emails from other people who have had the same experience.

I don't know why this is, but I do know that when you call a meter company to complain about a meter that is giving you wildly inaccurate or inconsistent readings, the customer service rep will always instruct you to do a control solution test, and that test will always be in range. So my cynical conclusion is that the only reason meters come with control solution is so that the meter company can avoid replacing defective meters.

I once had a meter so bad that the meter company recalled it and replaced it for free. The control solution test for that meter *still* came in within range.

So don't waste your valuable, overpriced strips on control solution tests.

Testing Hurts Am I Doing Something Wrong?

Poking yourself for a blood sugar test shouldn't have to hurt. The key is to find a really thin lancet and to change it rarely once it has been broken in. The lancets that come free with most blood sugar meters can hurt because they are too thick and may not launch to a consistent depth.

Fortunately, there is an alternative. I switched to the Accu-Chek Multiclix lancet many years ago and it is one of the few branded products I recommend. Those lancet needles are really thin and the device launches the needle really fast. The lancet and the cartridges it uses look really pricy when you see their box on the shelf—anywhere from $18 to $20. But lancet cartridges that come with the Multiclix lancet will last you for a decade or more. Why? Because the other secret of pain-free blood sugar testing is that you don't need to change your lancet more than once every three to six months.

This is not what the people who sell lancets tell you. But hey, their job is to sell lancets. Lancet companies display photos of used lancets taken under magnification that show huge chunks gouged out of their greatly magnified edges. Scary looking, but totally irrelevant. I learned long ago from the life-long Type 1s who frequented the old alt.support.diabetes newsgroup that it is perfectly safe and indeed much less painful to use an older lancet.

The only time you *do* have to change your lancet—immediately—is if someone else uses it. Using someone else's lancet is like using someone else's needle and can give you terrible blood borne diseases. No matter how much you trust someone, don't take the risk of sharing any kind of needle with them, including a blood sugar testing lancet.

Once you have gotten a thin lancet, you need to adjust the depth it reaches when you release it. This is usually is done by rotating a numbered collar to point to the proper number. Start with the lowest number, which is the shallowest. That one may not even break your skin. Then work your way up number by number until you reach the first setting that gives you a drop of blood big enough to provide a useful sample.

The next thing you need to do is change *where* you are testing. I don't know what imbecile decided people with diabetes would prefer to test on their arms, but whoever they were, they obviously don't have diabetes. It hurts more to test on your arms than it does on the proper location on your finger. Not only that, but readings taken from your arm are much less accurate than finger readings. Whoever came up with the arm testing idea must have been the same imbecile who decided that when testing using a finger you should point the lancet at the sensitive pad at your finger tip.

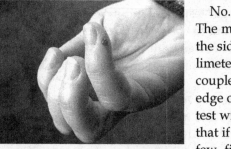

No. No. A thousand times no! The most painless place to test is on the side of your finger, a couple millimeters down from the top and a couple millimeters away from the edge of the nail. Some people like to test with different fingers, but I find that if I test in only a few spots on a few fingers, those fingers grow a little callus that makes the test even less painful. I usually test on the sides of my ring or pinky fingers.

I've also learned to take my lancet device with me to doctor's appointments, because my doctor's nurse often takes blood for in-office cholesterol or A1C tests. When he does, he pulls out one of those big railroad spikes and drives it—of course—into the sensitive pad of my finger tip. When I bring my own lancet and use it, with his permission, I can type without pain for the next two days after the appointment!

Can I Reverse Diabetes by Losing Weight?

It depends on how you define "reverse." If by that term you mean make your diabetes go away, so that you can eat whatever you want without it affecting your blood sugar, the answer is a resounding no. When I polled a group of highly motivated people with Type 2 Diabetes several times, asking them whether weight loss had had a significant impact on their blood sugars, only one or two said it had. The rest said that their blood sugars still responded to carbs the same way they had before they lost weight, even when they had lost a lot of it. That was my own experience, too, after I got down to a completely normal weight and maintained it for years.

But the whole weight loss thing is a red herring. You don't need to lose a pound to bring your blood sugars back to normal. Cut the carbs and the blood sugars come down no matter what you weigh.

And here is where it gets interesting. Because when people start following the strategy we'll be discussing in the next pages just to lower their blood sugar they also lose weight, even if they aren't consciously trying to limit their calories. Some of them lose a lot of weight. I have gotten emails from people—usually men—who report that much to their surprise they have dropped 50 to 70 lbs after getting their blood sugar under control. That much weight loss isn't typical, but most people will lose a few pounds as hunger levels drop dramatically when their blood sugars flatten out.

One reason doctors think that diabetes can be reversed—i.e. cured— by losing weight is that some of their less honest peers have made themselves very visible in the media with claims that their patients have, in fact, reversed their diabetes through weight loss achieved by eating the doctors' favorite, very extreme diet. But if you take the time to hunt down these studies and read the full text, you'll find one of two things: a) The definition of "reversing diabetes" turns out to mean "declaring people cured when their A1Cs are still over 7.5% or b) Describing a very low calorie diet as a "low fat" diet when it is also a very low carb diet and then confusing the dramatic lowering of blood sugar caused by eliminating hundreds of grams of carb with a cure, even though that "cure" goes away as soon as the subjects start eating carbs again.

What's the Best Diet for Diabetes?

Changing how you eat is the best way to lower your blood sugar. But if you have tried eating the typical "diabetes diet" that doctors and trained nutritionists suggest, you may have experienced dispiriting results. That's because these diets almost universally ignore the single most important fact about Type 2 Diabetes:

It's the carbs you eat that raise your blood sugar.

For decades trained dietitians have designed diabetes diets around the now debunked belief that eating fat causes heart attacks. Not only that, since people with diabetes so often have kidney disease, a second, also now debunked medical theory taught nutritionists that eating protein, too, would damage diabetic kidneys.

So what are you left with when you craft a diet for people with diabetes that contains almost no fat or protein? A diet packed full of carbohydrates—the same carbohydrates that gave these people their diabetic blood sugars to begin with.

Medical research published over the past 15 years has made it clear that it is perfectly safe to eat a most fats and that eating protein doesn't worsen kidney disease. You can review that research on this Blood Sugar 101 web page "Studies Proving The Safety and Efficacy of the Low Carb Diet" at **http://www.bloodsugar101.com/19066498.php** and on the Blood Sugar 101 web page "Diabetic Kidney Disease." **http://www.bloodsugar101.com/16351841.php#protein**..

So with that in mind, there is really only one diet fact you need to remember: **The best diet for someone with diabetes is a diet that keeps their blood sugars from rising after meals to the levels where diabetic complications and heart disease start to develop.**

For almost all of us, that diet will be a diet with a lot less carbohydrate in it. So I usually suggest that people start out by testing their blood sugar one or two hours after eating the meals they usually eat to see how high these meals are pushing their blood sugars. Then I tell them to try eating something similar with fewer carbs and see what impact that has on their post-meal blood sugars.

Cut carbs by doing things like taking the bun off your burger and topping it with tomatoes and some extra cheese. Skip the fries and have a small salad or pickles instead. Have ham and eggs for breakfast instead of cereal. Learn how to make protein pancakes and eat them instead of the flour versions. You'll find lots more suggestions on this webpage: What Can You Eat When You Are Cutting Carbs? You'll find it at **http://www.bloodsugar101.com/18856280.php**.

If you are like most people with diabetes, making changes like this will drop your blood sugar very quickly. Keep whittling way at how much carbohydrate you are eating until you can hit your blood sugar targets. This approach is so ridiculously simple my son suggested I title this section, "Massachusetts Woman Discovers One Weird Trick to Master Diabetes." But simple or not, it works. It doesn't matter if the carbs you cut are oatmeal and bananas or french fries and ice cream, the fewer carbs you eat of any description, the lower your blood sugar will be.

Once your post-meal blood sugar has dropped to a safe level, all you have to do is figure out how many grams of carbohydrate were in the meals that worked so well for you. Then keep eating meals that don't contain more carbs than that.

You won't have to keep testing after every meal, though you will want to keep testing occasionally to make sure you stay on track. You'll also want to test new foods or meals whose carbohydrate content you can't estimate, like those you eat in restaurants.

WARNING: If you are using insulin or one of the drugs that stimulates your pancreas to secrete insulin, you will need to cut your carbs slowly. If you remove them all at once you risk having a hypo, as your insulin dose was probably designed with the assumption that you are eating meals that are mostly carbs. As your blood sugar slowly drops you should be able to lower your insulin doses cautiously. If you are taking insulin-stimulating pills, you should be able to lower the dose or stop them entirely, too. But because insulin and insulin secreting drugs can cause dangerous hypos if you eat less carbohydrate than the dose was designed for, you will have to be more cautious.

If you don't know how to adjust your insulin dose, report your lowest blood sugars to whoever prescribed your insulin or pills and ask them to tell you how to safely lower your current dose.

The drugs that may make it unsafe to lower your carbs quickly besides insulin are the sulfonylurea and meglitinide drugs like glyburide, glipizide, glimepiride, repaglinide and nateglinide.

Metformin, Januvia, Victoza, won't cause hypos if you cut carbs. If you are taking Invokana or Jardiance, don't cut your carbs below about 110 grams a day, as these drugs may be dangerous if you take them while eating a ketogenic diet. (Discussed on Page 91.)

This 'Test, Test, Test" technique, where you use the feedback from testing the meals you eat to determine just how much carbohydrate your system can handle, is far more powerful than any of the commonly prescribed Type 2 Diabetes drugs. The drugs generally lower people's A1Cs by somewhere between .5% and 1%. But people who try this "Test, Test, Test" technique often write to tell me they've dropped their A1Cs by, 3, 5, or even 10 percentage points—from 16% to 6%. You can read the stories of people who have done this, written in their own words, on the 5% Club web page.

But you don't have to take their word for it—or mine, either. The beauty of this approach is that your trusty blood sugar meter will tell you within a few days whether this diet approach will work for you or not. Test how high a meal raises your blood sugar an hour or two after you have eaten. Then cut back on the carbs in that meal, and test it again. If your blood sugar drops, keep cutting down the carbs until you like what you see on your meter. That's all there is to it.

The one page flyer you'll find in the next section summarizes this strategy in a few easy steps. Download a copy and post it on the fridge. This flyer is my version of a message that a woman named Jennifer used to post on the alt.support.diabetes newsgroup when new people joined the conversation. Everyone who uses this strategy owes her a huge debt of gratitude!

Download at   http://www.bloodsugar101.com/how.php

How to Lower Your Blood Sugar

Step 1: Eat whatever you've been eating and write it all down

Eat normally, but use your blood sugar meter to test yourself at the following times. Write down what you ate and what your blood sugar results were:

Upon waking (fasting)

One hour after each meal

Two hours after each meal

Note: People often ask where to start measuring the hour after eating. For most people measuring from the end of the meal works well. If you take more than 45 minutes to eat your meal, measure from when you eat the course that contains the most starch and sugar.

What this will tell you is when your blood sugar is at its highest after your meal and how long it takes to drop back down. Most people also will see that all starches and sugars, even the ones that nutritionists tell us are "healthy" like whole grains and fruits can raise our blood sugars dramatically compared to fats and proteins.

Step 2: For the next few days cut back on your carbohydrates

Cut back on breads, cereals, rice, beans, any wheat products, potato, corn, and fruit. If you are eating gluten-free foods, stop eating anything designed to replace wheat-based foods, too. Get most of your carbohydrates from veggies. Test your modified meals using the same schedule above. See what impact you can make on your blood sugar by eliminating various high carbohydrate foods.

Be aware that some foods, like pasta or pizza, digest slowly, so you won't see a blood sugar spike one hour after eating or even, at times, two. But if you test pasta at four or five hours after eating, you may see a spike. The same is true of foods that contain the sweeteners used in "sugar free" foods sold as being good for diabetic diets. These often will produce a significant blood sugar spike an hour or two later than when you'd see the spike from regular sugar. If a food seems too good to be true, test another hour or two later.

The closer we get to non-diabetic readings, the greater chance we have of avoiding horrible complications.

Here are what doctors currently believe to be non-diabetic readings:

Fasting blood sugar under 100 mg/dl {5.5}

One hour after meals under 140 mg/dl {7.8}

Two hours after meals under 120 mg/dl {6.6}

If you can do better than this, go for it. At a minimum, The American College of Clinical Endocrinologists recommends that people with diabetes keep their blood sugars under 140 mg/dl {7.8} two hours after eating.

When you achieve normal blood sugar targets, you can start cautiously adding back carbohydrates, making sure to test after each meal. Stop adding carbohydrates as soon as you get near your blood sugar targets.

Recent studies have indicated that your "after meal" numbers are those most indicative of future complications, especially heart problems.

Step 3: Test, Test, Test!

Remember, we're not in a race or a competition with anyone but ourselves. Play around with your food plan. Test, test, test! Learn what foods cause blood sugar spikes and what foods cause cravings.

No matter what anyone tells you, if a food raises your blood sugar over the targets you are aiming for, that food should not be part of your diabetes food plan. Your blood sugar meter will tell you what the best "diabetes diet" is for your body. Use it and regain your health!

Why Do You Suggest Testing One And Two Hours After Eating?

These times were chosen because approximately one hour after eating is when most people will see their highest reading after eating. However, it is possible that you aren't "most people." So when you first start testing, if you see the same readings at one and two hours, you might want to do some testing at times in between to see if perhaps your blood sugar is peaking much later.

The other reason to favor this testing schedule is that the research linking classic diabetes complications and blood sugars always references one or two hour meal or glucose tolerance test results. While blood glucose coming in from a meal does not act quite the way a glucose test drink acts, a one or two hour meal test will give you figures that are still comparable to the numbers you see in research.

If your A1C is high enough to suggest that you are experiencing big spikes after eating—for example if it is over 6.5%—but you aren't seeing them when you test, it is possible they are occurring later than is the case with most people. Or it may not be there. The A1C test can be very inaccurate. Some people with higher than expected A1Cs have tested their blood sugars every few minutes with a device called a Continuous Glucose Monitor for days and have never seen any spikes that would justify the A1C test results they get. By the same token, some people's A1Cs are always lower than expected based on what they see on their home tests.

One reason for delayed blood sugar spikes is that your digestive tract may be more sluggish than is normal. This will make carby foods digest more slowly than expected. A sluggish digestion can be the result of diabetic neuropathy. You can read more about this symptom on Page 216. But there are many other issues that can also cause it.

A few foods are known to cause slow digestion and delayed blood sugar spikes, particularly pizza and dried pasta. Pizza may cause spikes an hour later or more than normal, and pasta can cause a spike four or five hours after you eat it. Sugar-free foods also cause delayed spikes. If you eat any of these, test them an extra hour after when you would usually test.

Should I Start Counting the Hour from the Start or End of the Meal?

Most people will see their blood sugar peak 75 minutes after they start eating.

How long a meal lasts can influence where that peak occurs. So can how fast what you ate digests. Though we are trying to test as close to that peak as possible, there is no need to become obsessively exact. As long as you are consistent with when you test, your testing will tell you what meals are working and which ones aren't.

Should I Worry About Spikes Half an Hour After I Eat?

Years ago I read a study that found that there was no correlation between blood sugar readings taken before an hour had passed after eating a meal and the likelihood of developing complications. Unfortunately, I haven't been able to find it again and not because I haven't looked.

So I wouldn't waste valuable strips testing my blood sugar until an hour or so after eating.

I'm Addicted to Carbs, How Can I Possibly Cut Them?

I often hear people say that they are "addicted to carbs." This is trendy, but it applies a very loaded term to the effect carbs have on us that really isn't justified.

When we are addicted to something, be it an illegal drug or an antidepressant prescribed by our family doctor, it's because our brains have become remodeled in ways that are very difficult to reverse.

This is not what happens when you find yourself in a state where you are dominated by a seemingly irresistible craving for carbs. That craving is rarely caused by damage to your brain. Instead, it occurs because your brain is performing exactly the way brains are supposed to. I have discussed this topic at much greater length in my book about low carb diets, but I'll give you the brief summary here of what makes you crave carbs so obsessively and how you can get rid of those cravings.

Your brain's major job is to stay alive. This requires that it always have a steady supply of glucose. Because this is a matter of survival—you can die in six minutes if your blood sugar drops to zero—the brain reacts very strongly to any suggestion that its precious glucose supply might be under threat.

One big hint that this might be happening is when the blood sugar drops very quickly. And guess what, those steep drops happen all the time when you are in the earlier stages of blood sugar deterioration. Your blood sugar surges after a meal, because you no longer secrete insulin right after eating like a normal person would. But you still make enough insulin to knock down that high very quickly during the next hour or two after you eat, which keeps your doctor from noticing something is wrong.

When this is happening you end up with what we call "rollercoaster blood sugars." You eat a bunch of carbs, and your blood sugar shoots up to 250 mg/dl {13.9}. Then an hour later, it crashes back to 150 mg/dl {8.5}. But your brain doesn't respond by thinking, "Well, 150 mg/dl is still pretty high, no problem here." Instead, it goes, "Help! Blood sugar plunging! Who knows where it will end!" and sends out a cascade of hormones that have one job: getting you to stuff your face with more carbs to force your blood sugar to soar back up again.

This is why the more carbs you eat, the more carbs you want. This may look or even feel like an addiction, but unlike addiction, this vicious cycle can be broken pretty easily. If you can flatten out your blood sugars for three days in a row, you will be amazed at how that obsessive need to eat just fades away.

Doing an Atkins-style diet for a few weeks may be the best way to break your "carb addiction." I don't recommend an Atkins-style "induction diet" for people with diabetes long term, because the carb intake it recommends is too hard for most people to keep eating past the initial few months. But a few weeks on one, where you start off with two weeks where you keep your daily carb intake as close to 20 grams a day as possible, will go a long way to curing any carb "addiction" you might think you have.

Once you figure out that carb cravings are just a sign your blood sugars are rising too high, you can start raising your carbs very cautiously every few days until are no longer eating an extremely low carb diet, but where the blood sugar peaks and valleys that occur after meals aren't steep enough to set your brain into panic mode.

Why Did the Nutritionist Say My Brain Won't Work If I Cut Carbs?

As was mentioned earlier, when we discussed blood sugar, your brain needs a non-negotiable amount of glucose to keep you alive. However, what many nutritionists don't seem to understand is that you can provide all the glucose your brain needs without eating a single gram of carbohydrate, as long as you eat enough protein. That's because your liver is able to convert 58%of the protein you eat into glucose if that glucose is needed. You only need about 100 grams of glucose a day to keep your brain going, so even if you were to eat no carbohydrates at all, you could get by eating another 172 grams of protein each day. But it is almost impossible to eat no carbs. Even people who think they aren't eating carbs are usually getting 10-20 grams. Most people eating very low carb, ketogenic diets are eating closer to 60 grams than 20. That means they only need to make up for that extra 40 grams of missing glucose. That would require that they eat another 69 grams of protein, which they could get from eating two servings of Greek yogurt and three ounces of chicken breast.

If you don't eat any extra protein, you won't die. Your liver will just strip protein from your muscles, including, perhaps, your heart muscle, which isn't healthy.

There is another interesting fact few nutritionists seem to be aware of. Your brain only needs those 100 grams of glucose for the first three weeks or so of a period when you are eating very little carbohydrate. After that period has elapsed, you only need 40 grams of glucose, as some of your brain cells will have switched to burning ketones. That's a little more than you'd find in 4 ounces of chicken breast. The biggest problem most people eating carb restricted diets run into isn't getting too little protein, but too much.

None of this is anything you need to worry about when you are eating more than about 100 grams of carbohydrate a day. If you are eating less, you should eat more protein for the first three weeks, but after that you only need to increase your protein intake by a modest amount.

You can learn exactly how much protein you need to eat using a handy calculator that you can find on the Blood Sugar 101 webpage "Calculate Your Ideal Nutrient Intake for Weight Loss or Maintenance," at **http://www.bloodsugar101.com/DietMakeupCalc.php**.

I Tried Cutting Carbs and My Blood Sugar Went Up

There is a very small group of people who, unlike the rest of us, will see their blood sugars go up when they cut carbs and replace those carbs with fat. This appears to be caused by specific genetic abnormalities, possibly ones similar to the gene that makes those specially bred diabetic lab rats experience high blood sugars when they eat fat. I have heard from three people over the years who have experienced this effect, one of whom I knew well enough personally to trust their report.

If you find that replacing carbs with fats raises your blood sugars after meals, you may find that you do better on a mix of nutrients similar to what is described in the book *The Zone Diet*. That would be diet made up of about 40% carbs 30% protein and 30% fat.

How Many Grams of Carb Do You Eat?

People often ask me what I eat as if this information could guide them to a safe, healthy diet. But it won't. What I eat is what works for me, but you aren't me. Your genes aren't like mine. You may not be the same size, age, or gender as I am. Your ancestors didn't come from where mine did so they didn't adapt to the diet mine adapted to. And most importantly, you may not be taking the same medications I take.

That's why there is no way to find out what combination of foods and medications will control *your* blood sugars except to get out your trusty blood sugar meter and test, test, test.

How Do I Figure out How Much Carbohydrate Is in a Meal?

Figuring out how much carbohydrate is in the food you eat will take some work at first, but after a few months it will become much easier.

To do it you'll need to get into the habit of looking up how many grams of carb there are in a serving of the foods you usually eat. This part is easy. If you are eating packaged foods, read the nutritional label. If you are cooking from scratch, and I hope you are at least some of the time, type in the name of the food and the word "carbs" into the Google search field on your phone, tablet, or computer browser. Up will pop the information you are looking for. For example, if you type in on Google search "whole wheat toast carbs" it will reply with the information that 1 slice contains 12 grams.

That's the easy part. But you're not done. Because as sure as God made little green apples, your slice of whole wheat bread does not weigh the 28 grams that Google tells you is the weight of "One slice." The nutritional label on the kind of whole wheat bread I buy says one slice weighs 46 grams, which is almost twice that generic 28 grams. So that tells you that the amount of carbohydrate is that actual slice of bread is closer to 20 grams than 12.

The nutritional panels on many products play games like this. Try weighing what you'd consider to be a reasonable portion of ice cream. Chances are it weighs twice as much as the portion the label defines. That means it also contains twice as much carbohydrate and calories than the label lists, too. (Does this start to explain why you never lost weight on your calorie counting diets?)

Average fruit and veggie weights are another area full of pitfalls, since they don't come with nutritional labels. Pieces of fruit can range in size from very small to huge, so a carb count for a "medium apple" tells you very little. Similarly, it's impossible for anyone but a trained butcher to estimate accurately how much a piece of meat might weigh without throwing it on a scale.

There is a solution to this problem. Buy yourself a food scale. You can order a very good one online for about $25. For the cost of a single cheap dinner for two you have just acquired what is, besides your trusty meter, the most useful diabetes control tool you will ever own.

Make sure your scale can easily switch from displaying ounce to displaying grams, since the nutritional values you will find listed may be given in either of those two units.

You can't weigh everything, especially when you are eating out. Luckily for you, the law now requires many chains to publish the nutritional information for their foods online. Just use Google to search for the restaurant or convenience store name and "nutritional info." For example, type in "Chipotle Nutritional Info" and up pops the information you need to figure out—roughly—what went into your avocado bowl. Just be aware that the portion size can be a factor here, too. If a published carb count looks too good to be true and doesn't come with a portion size, it probably is misleading. Every now and then, order take out and bring your portion home so you can weigh it on a scale. This will tell you how much faith you can put in a restaurant's nutritional info page.

What Should I Eat in Place of The Carbs I Cut?

Protein and fat are your alternatives when you start cutting back on carbs. The general rule of thumb is that the fewer grams of carb you eat, the safer it is to eat fat. So if you are eating a very low carb diet, you can eat surprising amounts of fat and still lose weight and see your cholesterol come down.

However, if you are eating a moderate carb-restricted diet which still contains a good 125 g of carbs a day or more, you should not overdo the fat.

The Blood Sugar 101ulator that you can find at http://www.bloodsugar101.com/DietMakeupCalc.php can be very useful for figuring out how much fat to eat. Tell it how many grams of carbs you are eating and it will suggest what is the healthiest balance of protein and fat based on your age, size, weight, and, if you know it, body fat percentage.

If you've been taught that all saturated fat is poison, it's helpful to know that that belief was grounded in badly designed research. Most of the research about "saturated fat" used diets filled with hydrogenated fats like Crisco, which are trans fats. Trans fats are not at all the same as naturally occurring saturated fats like butter fat. Trans fat is indeed terrible for your heart, which is why they were banned from processed foods. Oils used for frying are also unhealthy because high heat damages them and produces byproducts that are bad for us. But the story is very different for healthy natural saturated fats from nuts, dairy, and the meat of animals that have not been fed diets full of pesticides, herbicides, and artificial hormones. The evidence is accumulating that these saturated fats are actually very good for us.

So add some unprocessed cheese to your lunch. Using half and half in your coffee instead of milk eliminates quite a few grams of carbs and tastes better, too. Nuts are wonderful snacks, as are sunflower seeds in the shell. Treat yourself to some dark chocolate, too. The darker the chocolate the lower the carbs. Nibbling on a nice piece of high quality dark chocolate can be as satisfying as a chocolate cupcake without sending your blood sugar up into the danger zone for two hours or more.

Why Did My Doctor Tell Me to Eat Complex Carbs?

Doctors just pass on the standard diet advice promoted by nutritionists, and they love to recommend that people with diabetes eat a diet full of what they call complex carbs or "low glycemic" carbs. They will claim these don't raise your blood sugar as high as what are described as simple carbs, the so-called "white foods:" white bread, white potatoes, and white sugar.

This idea arose because people with normal blood sugar can maintain very flat blood sugars if they eat carbs that digest slowly. That's because they secrete normal amounts of insulin. But the reason that people with diabetes *have* diabetes is that they no longer secrete enough insulin to process big loads of blood glucose, whether it comes in fast or slow. So what happens when a person who is diabetic eats a food containing "slow" carbs is that they see a slightly later blood sugar spike that is pretty much the same height as they would see after eating the same number of grams of a faster-digesting carb.

The misplaced trust in "slow carbs" is why nutritionists long believed that pasta was the perfect food for people with diabetes. It spikes a couple hours after potatoes or bread would, but the nutritionists who came up with the concept of slow carbs only tested their effect on blood sugar one hour after eating, or, rarely, two. The spike from pasta can occur four or five hours after you eat it.

Some slow carbs may seem to work just fine for people whose diabetes is recently diagnosed, because they are still making considerable amounts of insulin. But every gram of carbs in the pasta you eat does eventually turn into glucose and when it does, your pancreas is going to have to come up with the insulin to handle it. This may make it tougher to make the insulin needed to cover your fasting blood sugar, which makes it go up.

As is true of any food you might consider eating, you can determine just how healthy it is by getting out your blood sugar meter and testing your blood sugar after eating it. If you don't see a spike when you eat a food that contains a lot of carbs, test at three or four hours after eating instead of one and two.

Do Carbs in Fruits and Veggies Count the Same Way as Carbs in Bread and Potatoes?

Many people count their carbs very carefully when they start working on lowering their blood sugar. This is very helpful—unless they take one look at the carb counts for fresh vegetables and decide to skip the tomatoes and carrots to make more room for some carby snacks.

This is a huge mistake. The carbs in non-starchy veggies rarely push your blood sugar up to the levels you see when you eat processed foods like potato chips, bread, or candy. Unlike the processed junk foods, non-starchy vegetables and even a few starchy vegetables like squash and sweet potatoes provide fiber, vitamins, minerals, and other important micronutrients in a form that is much more accessible to your cells than anything that comes in a supplement bottle, no matter how expensive.

Just as breast milk is better for babies than anything you can get in a can, eating the foods our species has evolved to eat over the past 10 million years is always better than swallowing chemicals in a capsule.

So keep those vegetables in your new, improved diet, eliminating only those that push your post-meal blood sugars too far out of bounds. Sometimes you can still fit a somewhat starchy vegetable into your diet simply by eating half of what you'd usually consider a normal portion.

Fruits are a bit more problematic. They have been bred to be much higher in sugar than the fruits we evolved to eat, and many of the most delicious fruits will send blood sugars surging. I went many years eating only the low carb fruits: strawberries, raspberries, blackberries, and the occasional slice of papaya. But over time I have found that I can often find undersized fruits at discount markets, like Trader Joe's or ALDI that are far kinder to my blood sugar than the big ones usually sold at supermarkets. If you are stuck with monster fruits, cut one in half and only eat part of it.

My body craves citrus so strongly in the winter that I have to assume it knows what its doing. So I figure a half or quarter serving of raw fruit here and there through the day, which doesn't cause a giant spike might be a good compromise. Stay away from cooked or blended fruits, like the ones you get in a smoothie. A lot of raw fruit can boil down or grate up to what seems like a pretty small serving.

Isn't Fructose Healthier than Glucose Because It's Fruit Sugar?

This belief is very common among people who are into "health food" but it is dangerously wrong.

Though fruits do contain some pure fructose most of them also contain a lot more sucrose—the white stuff you sprinkle into your coffee. But even if they were all fructose, they would not be healthy to eat. The idea that fructose is healthy arose because when you consume pure fructose it doesn't raise your blood sugar. Well of course it doesn't. The term "blood sugar" refers solely to blood *glucose*. But consuming a lot of fructose can make it much tougher to control you blood sugar control over time.

That's because the fructose you consume goes straight to your liver where it is converted into fat, some gets released into your blood-stream, raising your triglycerides, but if there's a lot it stays in your liver where it gets stored as liver fat.

It is possible that this accumulated liver fat makes the liver much more insulin resistant. Having an insulin-resistant liver will raise your post-meal blood sugars dramatically because it won't stop dumping glucose into the bloodstream when you have just eaten the way a healthy liver will. The rising insulin levels that follow a meal are what tell a healthy liver that there is no need to top up the glucose supply and get it to stop that glucose dumping. An insulin resistant liver keeps pouring unneeded glucose into your blood while the glucose from your meal is coming in, making the peak far higher.

When you get to where you have an enormous amount of stored up liver fat, things get worse. The liver can become inflamed and start damaging your liver. At that point you may be diagnosed with a condition called NAFLD (non alcoholic fatty liver disease). It isn't going to kill you, but if you keep on piling on that liver fat, eventually you end up with a more serious condition called NASH (non-alcoholic steato-hepatitis). NASH causes your liver to harden up and eventually stop working. When your liver quits on you, unless you get an immediate liver transplant you are all done.

Most people diagnosed with Type 2 have been eating a diet filled with table sugar before their diagnosis. Since half of each molecule of table sugar turns into a fructose molecule when it is digested, they already have already built up a large store of liver fat. So if *you* have eaten a very sugary diet until now, go easy on sugar and the sugary fruits that are full of fructose, even though pure fructose, when consumed doesn't your raise blood sugar.

Is Sugar Worse than Bread and Potatoes?

Before I answer this, let me say that I like stuff with sugar in it. I've gone months without eating it, but in the end, I always come back to sugar. I just do my best to make sure that when I eat stuff with sugar in it, I eat it in portions that my blood sugar can handle. That means no cupcakes with icing, but yes to an occasional homemade, low flour, dense chocolate brownie. I also eat quite a lot of 72% dark chocolate, and the occasional bonbon. So you won't get a "sugar is evil" rant from me.

But I've been working on controlling my carbs since 1998 and have a good grasp on how my blood sugar works and what it can and can't handle. If you are just starting out, you don't yet have that knowledge. So be very careful with sugar until you have your blood sugar under control. Sugar is the substance most people with abnormal blood sugars have the hardest hard time with, and when they eat too much, it can send them completely off the rails. So I usually suggest that people starting out avoid foods with white and brown sugar, honey, or any other caloric sweetener until they have had their blood sugar under control for several months. At that point an occasional treat is fine, as long as you stay away from the sugar bombs that make it impossible to hit your blood sugar targets.

If you have been sugar-free for a while, things will taste a lot sweeter when they have very little sugar in them. For example, after years of making homemade cocoa with artificial sweetener, I have started making it with the white sugar that tastes a lot better. But I only put about half a teaspoon of white sugar in. At most this is two or three grams of carbs. I can handle that.

Foods that are pure starch are actually a bit healthier for you than those that are pure sugar, only because pure starches like rice, potatoes, and bread don't contain the fructose that makes up half of every molecule of sugar and turns into liver fat. Some starchy foods contain useful vitamins and nutrients that sugary junk foods don't, though that doesn't earn them a free pass.

What About Natural Sugars like Honey, Agave Nectar, and Maple Syrup?

To determine how healthy these supposedly natural sugars might be, you need only look at how much fructose they contain. Ninety-nine percent of the sugar found in Maple syrup is sucrose, plain old table sugar. The rest is a mix of pure glucose and pure fructose. So Maple syrup is really no different, metabolically, than table sugar.

Honey has a higher proportion of fructose to glucose than sugar, though the exact amount varies from type to type. The National Honey Board reports that on average the sugars in honey are 38% fructose, 30% glucose, and 1% sucrose.

Agave Nectar has by far the worst sugar profile. The sugar in it can be as much as 70% fructose, or possibly more. Measurements are hard to come by.

Corn syrup is not a natural sugar. It's produced via chemical processes. How much fructose there is in it can vary. Some people believe that the increase in obesity is due to the use of high-fructose corn syrups instead of sugar.

Should I be Eating Sugar-Free Foods?

High on the list of entries in the Food Marketing Hall of Shame are the "Sugar Free" foods marketed as being perfect for people with diabetes. These are almost always foods in which sugar has been replaced by lab created molecules that are labeled "Sugar alcohols."

These won't make you drunk. They don't have anything in common with the kinds of alcohol found in beer or wine. They are synthesized starches made from highly processed corn syrup that are specially constructed so they take a much longer time to digest than does regular table sugar.

Because they digest slowly, these sugar alcohols game the tests that nutritionists use to see how high something raises blood sugar. That's because those tests only last one or two hours, while the most common sugar alcohols used in sugar-free foods, don't break down into glucose that shows up in your blood stream for *three* hours. Then they do show up and do raise your blood sugar, though not by quite as much as regular sugar. Nice trick, food manufacturers!

How much glucose a sugar alcohol turns into varies from one to another. Every gram of sorbitol, xylitol, maltitol, and lacitol eventually digests into two to three calories worth of carbohydrate. Since a gram of table sugar contains only four grams of carbohydrate, there really isn't all that much difference between the two substances, save that the sugar alcohol takes longer to get to your bloodstream.

Of all these, sorbitol seems to be the most legitimate when found in food, as it usually appears in very small quantities, two or three grams. Tiny breath mints, gums, and sugar free maple syrup with a small amount of sorbitol can pacify your sweet tooth without raising your blood sugar. However maltitol and lacitol are often added in much larger quantities to foods—anywhere from 20 to 30 grams per serving. This can turn into a non-trivial amount of glucose.

Still, if this were the only thing going on with "Sugar free" foods, they would not have landed in the Hall of Shame. That happened because the "Sugar free" label is also applied to a shelf full of bakery products like muffins, cookies, and sweet breads. The number of grams of carbohydrates in these foods is extremely high, since they are all full of starchy flour. The carb counts are so high, in fact, that the companies that sell this stuff often define a "serving" on their nutritional labels as being one half of the food item.

So you might glance at the label of a sugar free muffin and think, "Hmmm. This only contains 25 grams of carbs, no big deal. That's not much more than a slice of bread." But the serving size, displayed in tiny print is "1/2 muffin" so the whole muffin (and we are not talking a big muffin, either) is actually 50 grams of carbs, which is enough to send most people's blood sugar up into the higher realms.

There is so much starch in these "sugar free" foods that if you are going to have yourself a muffin or donut you might as well eat the real thing. There is very little difference in the carb count, and the sugar free stuff tastes weird.

There is one last issue that may keep you from embracing "sugar free" foods full of sugar alcohols. While they do get digested into glucose in many of us, that doesn't happen for everyone or with every sugar alcohol. Apparently you need to be able to produce certain enzymes to be able to digest maltitol and lacitol, and what happens if you don't have those enzymes isn't pretty. In that case, these lab created, weirdo starch molecules make their way undigested into your lower intestine where they produce diarrhea so dramatic that after eating one serving of a food that contains them I guarantee you will never eat another one again. That last statement isn't based on hearsay. I apparently lack the enzyme needed to digest the lacitol found in sugar free ice cream. So as far as I'm concerned, giving children maltitol and lacitol-laced sugar free candy at Halloween is child abuse.

The one sugar alcohol that manages to pull off the trick of not digesting into glucose or turning into Ex-lax is erythritol. It has a strange kind of cool taste, but is delicious in chocolates. Unfortunately, it's expensive, so there are no longer any erythritol-sweetened chocolates on the market. I used to love them when there were. You can still buy bags of erythritol crystals at health food markets, at about $10 for a pretty small bag. But it doesn't work when you use it to try to sweeten hot drinks, as its sweetness completely disappears in cocoa or tea. I have found it works very well in baked goods where using a mix of half Splenda-sweetened sugar-free syrup and half erythritol crystals can be quite tasty.

Are Artificial Sweeteners Safe?

I get asked this a lot, because years ago there was a group of fanatics who spread rumors throughout the online world suggesting that artificial sweeteners were poison. This was uttered in the breathless tones of pure conspiracy theory with the usual claim that "the government doesn't want you to know..." all the dreadful things they claimed these sweeteners could do.

It is true that some of the older artificial sweeteners, saccharine and cyclamate were linked to cancer in rodent studies many decades ago. The evidence was not convincing enough for the FDA to ban saccharine, which is still found in the little pink packets used to sweeten coffee. The FDA did ban cyclamates in the United States though they continue to be sold in many other countries. I'm old enough to have drunk a lot of diet sodas sweetened with cyclamates and remember them as tasting much better than those made with aspartame.

Aspartame has been subjected to a great deal of scientific scrutiny due to the conspiracy theories that grew up around it. The evidence doesn't seem to support any of the wilder conspiracy claims. Some people say it gives them headaches. I think it tastes horrible, rather like licking a metal pipe, but apparently this is only the case if you have certain taste bud genes.

Sucralose (Splenda) is a newer artificial sweetener that has also attracted its share of conspiracy theorists. Again, the studies used to support their claims appear to be poorly designed and of questionable value. Back in the late 1990s, before Splenda was approved in the United States some of us in the online diabetes community used to mail order Splenda from abroad because it tasted so much better than the aspartame that was all that was available for calorie-free sweetening back then. I have consumed quite a bit of it over the years and found it did not, as is sometimes claimed, have a negative effect on my attempts to lose weight. Splenda is the only calorie free sweetener that you can cook with and have your foods turn out tasting sweet. The others get nasty when subjected to baking temperatures.

Stevia is the newest of the non-caloric artificial sweeteners. It is pitched as being a more "natural" sweetener since it is derived from an herb, but it takes a huge amount of chemical processing to turn a green leaf into a pure white powder. So this "natural" claim is pure marketing malarkey. You can get real stevia leaves in health food stores, though they aren't anything most people would want to have floating around in their coffee.

Stevia has a much shorter history than the other sweeteners and there is some evidence that it might promote cell mutation at higher doses, so given a choice, I would choose Splenda over stevia. However, as is the case with aspartame, the taste of stevia is greatly influenced by your taste bud genes. It doesn't taste sweet to me at all, though apparently it does to other people. You can't bake with stevia. It loses its sweetness when exposed to heat.

Some people report that their blood sugar rises when they use artificial sweeteners, especially Splenda. Researchers have also reported that when extremely obese, non-diabetic people consumed Splenda both their blood sugar and their insulin levels rose. But most people in the diabetes community who test their blood sugar regularly have *not* observed this effect. You can determine if it applies to you by testing your blood sugar after consuming a food or drink containing a lot of Splenda. Choose a drink other than coffee, as plain caffeinated coffee can raise blood sugar all on its own by stimulating the release of stress hormones.

Do Artificial Sweeteners Stop Weight Loss?

Some research has suggested that consuming sodas made with artificial sweeteners makes people gain weight because their sweetness stimulates some sweetness receptors in the gut and brain that make them expect sugar to be coming in. This could cause a normal person to secrete enough insulin to push their blood sugar low enough to result in a reactive hypo, which would, in turn make them very hungry.

Those who argue that artificial sweeteners make us fat point to studies proving that consumption of artificially sweetened sodas doesn't produce weight loss in women. These studies explain this is true because most women who consume diet sodas don't cut back on eating other sugary foods. It is also possible that the metabolic confusion caused by those stimulated sweetness receptors might also be driving their hunger for sugar.

Since news of these studies hit the airwaves, I've gotten a lot of questions from readers about whether using artificial sweeteners like Splenda will prevent weight loss. My answer is, as so often is the case, "It depends."

I know plenty of people who have lost significant amounts of weight and kept it off while consuming a lot of Splenda sweetened foods and drinks. I sure did. But these are also people who were carefully counting their carbs and keeping them quite low. When carbs are kept low, hunger is usually easy to control.

But if ordering a diet soda makes you feel like you've done what you need to do to be virtuous so now you can tuck into that plate of cookies without guilt, you do have a problem. It's also possible that when diet sodas are consumed along with enough carbs to create the kind of blood sugar spike that leads to hunger they may intensify the effect. It's hard to say.

The smartest thing to do is what you should be doing with anything you eat or drink. Try it and observe what happens in your own highly unique body after you consume it. For example, I learned years ago that I always got hungry after eating tiny breath mints containing sorbitol even though they only had a gram of carb in them. I could put Splenda in cup after cup of homemade cocoa and feel completely satisfied afterward, but those breath mints were something else entirely.

It's also worth noting that most sugar free soft drinks contain significant amounts of caffeine. This may also explain why they make some people hungry. It also may explain why some people report that artificial sweeteners raise their blood sugar. Caffeine alone can raise blood sugar by stimulating the release of stress hormones.

Should I Eat a Lot More Protein when I Cut Carbs?

Unless you are cutting your carbs down to less than 100 grams a day you should not eat any more protein than usual. And even when you are eating fewer than those 100 grams of carb a day, the amount of protein you actually need is far less than most people eating low carb diets tend to consume.

If you are trying to lose weight on a low carb diet, eating too much protein will stall weight loss. It can even raise your fasting blood sugar, since roughly half of the protein you eat can be converted into glucose by your liver. Eating too much protein can also make your urine full of irritating ammonia and cause bad breath.

Use the nutritional calculator you'll find on the Blood Sugar 101 website to determine what is the proper amount of protein to eat. That amount should be one that provides just enough protein to build and maintain healthy muscle and to provide some extra protein for the liver to convert into glucose when you're eating at an extremely low carbohydrate intake level. As your carb intake rises, the calculator will shift the intake it recommends to one that matches the Zone Diet. That diet was found to be the healthiest of the moderate-carb diets studied in a large, two year comparison study

What Fats Do You Recommend?

Because I believe that it is important not to get too obsessional about the food we eat, I try not to go overboard or ever suggest that people have to eat some ideal, utterly perfect diet. But if you are going to eat more fats to replace some of the calories you got rid of when you cut down on your carbs, it really matters that the fats you eat not be the damaged fats, heart-unfriendly fats, or contaminated fats found in so much packaged food.

One of the biggest problems with the faddy ketogenic diets that were popular 20 years ago is that people who ate them so often ended up eating a lot of very salty processed food that was full of MSG and very damaged fats. So when you think fat, don't think bacon, hot dogs, or fast food burgers without buns. You'd do a lot better eating better quality meat, poultry, and seafood you cook yourself, unprocessed cheeses without additives and stabilizers, nuts and nut butters without added sugar, and additive free dairy products. When in doubt, read the label. If a product has a long list of unnatural sounding additives, they aren't good for your diet.

Here is a handy reference to help you sort out the good and bad fats:

GOOD FATS

Butter, Cheese, Cream and Half and Half

Recent research has validated what my butter loving body always knew, that butter is both delicious and healthy. If you can afford it, organic is better, because so many pesticides and herbicides are fat soluble and end up in the body fat of the animals that eat them. That said, I've mostly eaten conventional dairy products over the past decades and I'm still alive.

Cheese forms a major part of my own diet as I'm not all that fond of big chunks of meat, am burnt out on chicken, and can't stand the taste of most fish. The cheeses I prefer are the European ones you can get at Trader Joes, or if they aren't available, plain cheddars, swiss, brie, and cream cheese.

I avoid processed cheeses as they are often filled with starch, flavorings, and the inorganic phosphates which promote the formation of plaque in your arteries and damage marginal kidneys (see Page 117). However, there is no need to get crazy about this. A slice of American cheese won't kill you. But make it an occasional slice, not a daily habit.

Olive Oil

This is often recommended by dietitians. Unfortunately, most of the olive oil you buy in the United States is not what the label claims it is, and it may be adulterated by the addition of cheap, highly processed vegetable oils. I must confess that when someone gave us what was supposed to be the very expensive pure, grove-sourced virgin olive oil some years ago, I found the taste very harsh, so it's likely true that most of what we think is olive oil is much less flavorful cheaper oils. I occasionally cook with the stuff from supermarket shelves when I make foods that go well with olive oil. But mostly I cook with butter and coconut oil.

Coconut Oil

This is a current faddy wonder food. I reviewed the research that is supposed to back up the claims that it has magical weight loss properties, back when I wrote my book, *Diet 101*, and was underwhelmed. There is no convincing evidence coconut oil boosts metabolism or improves weight loss. So don't go adding it to your diet, on top of what you usually eat thinking it will enhance fat burning. The research suggests that if it does help at all in weight loss it only does so when it replaces other oils calorie for calorie. Even then, the difference it makes is tiny.

However, coconut oil is a very good oil to cook with in situations where butter would burn. You can make a delicious refrigerator fudge with coconut oil and cocoa or bakers' chocolate by melting them together and adding your favorite sweetener. Put it in the fridge to harden, and enjoy.

Vegetable Oil in Modest Amounts

The only vegetable oils I eat are those that come in bottled salad dressings and restaurant foods. I don't cook with them. This isn't because I'm fanatical. I just like the taste of the other cooking fats and oils listed above better. Over the years, bottle after bottle of canola oil has gone rancid in my pantry because I've never used it. So finally I got smart and stopped buying it. The science suggests that most of the vegetable oils aren't particularly good for us, due to their high Omega-6 oil content.

Cocoa Butter

Dark chocolates made only with the natural fat of cocoa butter are a wonderful treat that is completely safe and healthy. Read labels and avoid the stuff which is full of added vegetable oils instead of this cocoa butter. Recently palm oil has been sneaking into our chocolate supply which is very bad news for our health.

Nut Oils

These are healthy when eaten in the form of the actual nuts. Peanut oil may not be all that good for you if you consume a lot of it. Untreated nut oils need to be eaten quickly as they do go rancid.

Fish Oil

I take a capsule of this nasty-tasting stuff every day, simply because it keeps my eyes from drying out when our radiators make my house feels like the Sahara each winter. But the evidence for fish oil having a healthy effect on your heart hasn't held up to scrutiny. Still, it is useful stuff if you have the dry eye problem that many of us older people and postmenopausal women deal with.

The problem with eating fish oils that come from actual fish you eat is that all the fish you can buy now are so heavily contaminated with mercury and other toxins that fill our seas that it isn't wise to eat very much of them. When you look up how much mercury is supposed to be in a species of fish, most of the values you will find turn out to come from databases that haven't been updated since the 1970s. When scientists nowadays catch fish and measure how much mercury is in what they caught, it is usually alarmingly high—far higher than what the only available statistics suggest it would be.

So ignore the advice about how healthy fish is and consume it sparingly. I know two people whose daily fish habit led them to develop mercury poisoning and led to them having to undergo potentially hazardous chelation treatment performed by mainstream doctors.

Supposedly the fish oil capsules I buy at the drug store have been purified of mercury, but given my distrust of unregulated supplement manufacturers I don't trust this label claim and only take one capsule a day.

BAD FATS

Trans Fat

Back when I first got diagnosed with diabetes in 1998, trans fat was present in just about any processed food you could buy. The book *Protein Power* turned me on to just how bad trans fat was, and I started reading labels and not bringing home foods that contained them. This was a good call. Trans fat was eventually proven to be so bad for our arteries that it was eventually banned. Even so, it still appears in a surprising amount of packaged food.

The loophole is that the law allows food manufacturers to put trans fat into a food as long as that food contains less than a gram of trans fat per serving. However, as you may recall, the serving sizes listed on the label is often much smaller than the portion size a normal person would eat. So you are likely to be getting more of it than you realize when you consume normal, real world portions. And beyond that, there is also a ton of evidence that food companies lie on their labels, since the FDA does not have the resources to check that products actually contain what their labels say they do.

Still, the FDA states that no amount of trans fat is safe. Given the dangerous garbage they approve, I have to assume this stuff must be really ugly. So read labels and don't bring home anything with trans fat listed in the ingredients. This means anything that uses the term "hydrogenated" when referring to a fat or oil.

Palm Oil and Palm Kernel Oil

When trans fat was banned, the food industry rushed to replace it with various forms of oil derived from tropically grown palm trees. They did this because these palm oils don't go rancid and can sit on a store shelf for decades without a change in flavor.

The first time I tasted something made with one, I noticed that it clung to my lips like lip gloss rather than melting like butter or even the old trans fat. I found it hard to believe that any fat that didn't melt at body temperature could possibly be good for me. So I have been avoiding it when possible ever since.

Even if my reasoning turns out to be faulty, it looks like I made a good call. The European Food Safety Authority (EFSA) said in May of 2016 that palm oil generates more of a potentially carcinogenic contaminant than other vegetable oils do when that palm oil is refined at temperatures above 200 degrees Celsius (392 degrees F.), which is a common practice. As a result the EFSA is now threatening to ban palm oil.

The effects of highly processed palm oils on the heart haven't been investigated yet, but I wouldn't be surprised if this stuff also turned out to be worse than trans fat in terms of promoting heart disease. Palm oil production is also devastating to our environment because vast tropical regions are being clear cut to grow the short-lived trees that produce it.

Health food stores often sell foods with palm kernel oil as if this were better for you, and may explain it is a traditional food in some African cultures. But the real palm oil that is eaten in some cultures in Africa and elsewhere is orange and has a strong taste. If yours is clear or white, it has been processed and is no longer the same stuff.

Should I Be Eating Organic Food Only?

If you can afford to eat all organic foods, it's a good idea to do so, given the high amount of pesticides and herbicides in conventionally farmed foods. These chemicals have been shown in study after study to increase insulin resistance and harm beta cells. People who eat a lot of animal meat, in particular, should think twice before eating the fat of animals raised in environments full of these toxins.

That said, I've been able to keep my blood sugar under control for decades eating mostly conventional foods, so don't agonize about it if you can't avoid eating them.

Should I Be Eating Gluten-Free?

Eating a gluten free diet won't in and of itself lower your blood sugar unless you have celiac disease, the condition where consuming gluten leads to system-wide inflammation. Nor will eating a gluten-free diet lower your blood sugar if you replace wheat and corn with equally starchy rice and tapioca flour. Unless you have a true intolerance to wheat gluten that results in inflammation, a carb is a carb, no matter what plant it comes from.

But eliminating gluten from your diet can be very helpful if you have an ongoing problem with heartburn that is severe enough that you are taking pills for it every day. Heartburn often disappears within days once you cut gluten out of your diet. Since evidence is accumulating that chronic use of all kinds of heart burn drugs increases the chances that you will develope dementia, getting off those pills may make a huge improvement in your health.

If you find you feel better when you cut out gluten, it may also make it much easier to avoid eating the many seductive wheat-based junk foods that are such a temptation to those of us trying to cut down on carbs.

My own experience with this has been that after avoiding all foods containing flour for a few years I recovered my ability to eat it without experiencing heartburn. However, when I started eating more wheat, it came back some years later.

Will Cinnamon Lower My Blood Sugar?

No. But there's no harm in eating it. Cinnamon was the cure *du jour* back in the early 2000s. It's been thoroughly debunked, but still promoted by the usual sleazy online supplement sellers.

Some of these shysters claim that their cinnamon will lower your blood sugar because it's an exotic variety that isn't the same stuff you find in the $1 bottles sold at the Dollar Store. This is misleading. The now debunked studies that were believed to prove that cinnamon lowered blood sugar were done with the exact same cheap stuff sold in the grocery store.

What About Apple Cider Vinegar?

The idea that drinking apple cider vinegar can cure all that ails you was heavily promoted in the 1980s by serial fraudster, Kevin Trudeau. There is no basis to his claims but they still sell a lot of apple cider vinegar.

What little evidence there is suggests that drinking vinegar might make a tiny improvement in your blood sugar, but the quality of the research is so poor and the improvement that vinegar is reported to make is so tiny that there is no reason to use vinegar of any kind for anything except a piquant salad dressing that makes your greens more appetizing.

As is the case with anything that claims to lower blood sugar, you don't need to take my word for it. Just test it at home with your meter.

If it works for you, great!

Where Can I Find Good Recipes and Ideas for What to Eat?

People with diabetes vary so greatly in terms of what they can eat and still reach their blood sugar targets that it's tough to make recommendations. I bought a bunch of low carb cookbooks back when I started working on my own blood sugar, but I never ended up cooking any of the recipes I found in them. Many were for dishes that were just too different from the kinds of foods I like to eat. Some used weird substitutions that didn't work for me. Others required expensive, perishable, exotic ingredients that I never had handy when it was time to make dinner. Some had far more carbs than I could handle when the portion size was large enough to make me feel like I'd had a meal.

I did learn quite a few helpful tricks from people who used to post on the old alt.support.diet.low-carb newsgroup. Their recipes are at **https://www.camacdonald.com/lc/LowCarbohydrateCooking-Recipes.htm**. Another useful website is "Linda Sue's Low Carb Recipes and Menus" at **http://genaw.com/lowcarb/recipes.html**.

But after all these years, mostly what I eat is the same stuff I used to eat, but with much smaller portions of the carby stuff. I also eat more meaty soups and low carb veggies. I now use one slice of bread to make a sandwich, not two. I nibble at pizza crust and then mostly just eat the topping. Half a small new potato works for me, though a big baked one doesn't. The chili we eat at our house is light on beans and full of chopped up veggies. I make macaroni and cheese without the macaroni using a serving of polenta to line the baking dish and adding lots of mushrooms and chicken breast to fill it up.

But that's me. What is most likely to work for you will be versions of the foods *you* are used to eating that replace high carb ingredients with something your body can handle better.

One last thought: Whatever you enjoy eating, you'll do infinitely better over the years if you learn how to cook the foods you enjoy at home from scratch. The foods you make will be so much more delicious than what you buy in a box, bag, or can. They will also be free of the many additives that pollute all supermarket prepared foods.

Chapter Four

Should I Eat Dr. _____'s Diet?

What Do You Think of Dr _____'s Diet?

My strongly held belief is that you will do best eating the diet you customize by cutting carbs out of the foods you already like to eat. That's because you are much more likely to *stick to* that kind of diet. We are going to have diabetes for the rest of our lives, which we hope will be long ones. So the diet we use to control our blood sugars has to be one we really can keep eating for decades to come. No faddy diet fills that requirement, no matter what it does to our weight or blood sugar in the short-term.

But every few years a new doctor comes out with a diet book that gets him the TV appearances that turn his book into a bestseller. These books always promise that some brand new, easy to understand, but peculiar "diet secret" will heal your diabetes and make you as good as new. The attention these fad diets get lead to my getting a lot of letters from people who ask me what I think about these doctors and their diets.

Well, since you asked, I think too many of these authors are exploitative opportunists who don't care how many people's health they hurt as long as they get rich. Of the few who aren't out to make a buck, too many are fanatics driven by extreme political views or an obsessive belief that there is one single solution that will cure everyone no matter what their problem.

Harsh words, yes. But with the millions these doctors have made selling their magical cures, you'd expect to find at least a handful of people online enthusing about how their blood sugars are now perfect after eating one of these magical diets. But you don't. And there is a reason for this.

Almost none of the doctors who put their names on such a book have any professional experience treating people with diabetes. A quick look at the MDs whose books are usually at the top of the diabe-

tes bestseller list on reveals only one who was trained in endocrinology — Dr. Richard K. Bernstein — and his book has never been the kind
of bestseller that shows up in Walmart.

Of the rest of the MDs who have written bestselling diabetes books,
several never made it through their residencies, which means they
have never actually practiced medicine. This describes Dr. Mosley of
5:2 fast diet fame and Dr. Neal Barnard, the professional vegan.

Dr. Mosley's understanding of diabetes is so out of date that in his
5:2 diet bestseller he claimed to have reversed his own diabetes by
dropping his fasting blood sugar below 140 mg/dl {7.8}. That was the
diagnostic level used to diagnose diabetes from fasting blood sugar
until 1997. But it changed to 125 mg/dl {7.0} in 1998. He was still citing
that level in his book published 15 years later n 2013. That no one
picked up this error while the book was in production should make
you realize that editors of this kind of book do zero fact checking for
any of the claims made. It is strictly a case of "Trust me, I'm a doctor."

Dr. Barnard, another huge bestseller, trained as a psychiatrist but
has never practiced, having dedicated his life to running a PETA-
affiliated, deceptively titled organization, "The Physicians Committee
for Responsible Medicine" (PCRM). PCRM is an extreme animal rights
group, only 5% of whose members are physicians. It's mission is to try
to convince the public that all non-vegan diets are harmful. It has a
history of doing this by producing false news.

Dr. Barnard bases his claim that he can cure diabetes with a strict
vegan diet on a study which includes his name in its list of authors,
though Dr. Barnard, another non-practicing MD, does not have any
official position where he would have access to his own lab or a team
of researchers. What his oft-cited study actually found was that people
who ate his vegan diet for a year and a half (72 week) lowered their
A1Cs from an average of 8.0% to an average of 7.77%. Thus they
ended up with an average blood sugar of 177 mg/dl {9.8}. Only someone who cares more about saving animals than healing people could
describe this as "reversing diabetes."

Dr. Joel Fuhrman, the current top diabetes cure huckster, is also a
torchbearer for the vegan cause and a member of Dr. Barnard's PCRM.
To his credit, at least Dr. Fuhrman appears to actually have a medical
practice. But there is no reason to believe his vegan cure would be any
more effective than Dr. Barnard's.

Dr. Julian Whitaker's bio states he dropped out of a surgical resi-
dency to become an "alternative health practitioner." That term means
whatever the person using it wants it to mean. He claims to be board
certified as an alternative health practitioner, but the board he was

certified by is not a medically recognized board. It is likely to be one of many vanity organizations that will certify anyone who has earned an MD degree if they pay a fee. Dr. Whitaker has written diet books claiming to cure a wide variety of chronic illnesses, which is always a bad sign.

Among the diet book authors who do have legitimate medical credentials, you will find quite a few cardiologists. Most people don't realize it, but cardiologists get no training in nutrition or in how to treat diabetes. That is the job of the primary care physician or the endocrinologist. A cardiologist's interaction with people with diabetes is limited to testing their heart function and doing surgical procedures like installing stents.

Nevertheless, some of the top earning authors of bestselling diet and diabetes books have been cardiologists, including Dr. Robert Atkins, Dr. William Davis, and Dr. Agatston author of the South Beach Diet. Their diets are better than those of the fanatics and hucksters, but none of them has much insight into diabetes, and they tend to write assuming that cutting carbs is all someone with diabetes needs to do. It very often isn't.

Some of these doctors who have written diet books claim to have treated many thousands of patients in diet clinics. But if they have, these patients are suspiciously silent about their experiences. The exception is Dr. Bernstein. You can find quite a few people online who have actually been treated by him at his office. He is a stellar exception to the rule that doctors who write about diabetes don't know squat about it.

Should I Be Eating a Ketogenic Diet?

If you cut your carbohydrate intake below a certain, very low level, your body will switch from burning glucose for most cellular operations to burning ketones. These are substances derived from the breakdown of fats: both the fats we eat and those stored in our body fat. As the ketone levels in your blood and urine rise on an ultra low carb diet, your diet can now be described as a "ketogenic diet."

The Atkins Diet is the best known and oldest of the ketogenic weight loss diets, though the description of the diet given in the books that carry his name have changed over the decades. Dr. Richard K. Bernstein's diabetes diet is also a ketogenic diet. However, unlike most doctors who write about ketogenic diets, Dr. Bernstein has an encyclopedic knowledge of what it takes to treat diabetes and does not fall into the trap of thinking that diet is the solution to every blood sugar problem.

Ketogenic diets will drop your blood sugar like a stone. They are a very good way to "detox" from eating too much mindlessly consumed high carb junk food. But most people with diabetes find them too hard to stick to over the decades that they will have to eat an effective diabetes diet. If the only diet that will lower your blood sugar to normal levels is a ketogenic diet you will have two choices. One is to stick with it, even when you start to burn out. The other is to eat the diet as long as you enjoy eating it but then ask your doctor for a safe drug or two if you start seeing burnout looming ahead.

What Makes a Diet Ketogenic?

The daily carbohydrate intake at which a diet becomes ketogenic, which I call "the ketogenic boundary," differs from person to person. It's higher for people who are very large and lower for us smaller, older people, especially females.

For me, that boundary is set at 70 grams a day. If I eat under that level, within a few days I start peeing ketones, which you can sometimes smell and always verify with the ketone test strips you can buy at the drug store.

On the way to making the switch from burning glucose to burning ketones, your body burns through a cache of stored glucose it keeps in your liver and through smaller deposits of stored glucose found in your muscles. This glucose is stored in the form of a substance called glycogen. Glycogen is heavy because there is a lot of water bound up in it. So when you burn it off you lose a couple pounds very quickly and pee your brains out, too because all the water stored along with that glycogen gets released. This makes people feel instantly skinny and makes them think that if they keep eating low carb diets they will drop the same three to twelve pounds they lost in the first week of their diet for months to come—which they won't.

If you keep your carb intake below that ketogenic boundary you will not store any more glycogen and will stay slimmer. But the day you eat enough carbs to go over that boundary, the glycogen fills right back up, bringing with it all that heavy water. You'll wake up three to twelve pounds heavier, which can be quite upsetting if you don't understand what just happened.

Some people who are a lot larger than I am, and/or male, have a much higher ketogenic boundary. They drop into a ketogenic state while eating 100 grams of carbs a day or more. They may also lose a lot more scale weight over the first few days of a ketogenic diet than the two or three pounds I'll lose because their livers store a lot more glycogen.

Note, however, that I called it "scale weight." You should never confuse this easy come easy go weight loss or gain with body fat loss or gain. You lose body fat on a ketogenic diet only if you eat less calories than you need, as is true with all other diets. Though it is true that people with diabetes tend to lose more fat on ketogenic diets than other diets because they produce the flat blood sugars that eliminate hunger. The absence of sugar from these diets may also be a factor here too.

If you are limiting carbs to keep your blood sugar healthy, you will want to decide whether or not you want to eat a ketogenic diet. If not, set your daily carb intake high enough so you don't go up and down over your ketogenic boundary. If you do, the continual weight gain and weight loss can be quite unpleasant. Fasting diets also can get you burning off glycogen and peeing your brains out on the days you fast, though the glycogen comes back after you eat normally the next day.

Why Can't I Lose Weight on a Ketogenic Diet?

Ketogenic diets can produce dramatic weight loss in some lucky people. But there is a reason the most vocal enthusiasts for the ketogenic diet online are male, many of them males who at one time were very large. Women may find a ketogenic diet much harder to live with long term, and anyone who spends any time reading low carb diet forums will quickly notice that most of the women who eat these diets for any significant amount of time stall out at weights way above their goal weight.

The reason for this is that, despite what you will read in the books written by the men who get rich pitching the ketogenic diet as a cure-all, calories matter in ketogenic diets just as much as they do in any other diet. And women need far, far, fewer calories than men do.

Where this causes a problem unique to ketogenic diets is that the most satisfying ketogenic diets seem to be ones where the dieter eats a great deal of fat along with enough protein to build and repair muscle and to provide the raw material from which the liver can synthesize the small amount of glucose that the brain requires to function.

But women's smaller calorie allowance means they can't eat a whole lot of satisfying fat on a calorie-limited ketogenic diet before hitting their calorie limit. This is even truer if they are eating enough protein to repair and maintain their muscles.

A large, male, ketogenic dieter can easily eat a diet that is 80% fat, which is the level at which most enthusiasts who post online report they lose weight most easily and are free of hunger. Most women who are consuming enough protein to avoid cannibalizing muscle—which could be dangerous to their heart muscles—will not have enough calories left to be able to eat a diet that is more than 69% fat. And the closer they get to their goal weight, the less fat they can eat, because, of course our calorie needs drop dramatically as we lose weight.

So women who embark on ketogenic diets hoping to lose a lot of weight need to carefully count their calories and go easy on portion sizes. Not for us are the 18 oz steaks and dollops of blue cheese dressing beloved by the large male keto-bloggers. Too much fat, even though it won't raise blood sugar, will stop weight loss cold.

Ketogenic diets are useful for weight loss when they do control your hunger, though most of us will have to keep an eye on those calories. One worked very well for me when I carefully counted my calories when I was in my 50s. But now that I am nearing 70, eating one for more than a few weeks leaves me feeling drained of energy so I only eat ketogenic diets every now and then when I feel like carb creep is getting out of hand and want to break some bad carb-centered habits.

Why Is My Weight Going Up and Down a Couple Pounds Every Day?

Eating too close to your ketogenic boundary can do this, as discussed earlier. The other thing that causes this kind of intense day to day fluctuation is eating lots of salt and/or MSG.

I have learned over the years that every time I eat lunch at my favorite Chinese restaurant, even if my blood sugar is perfect for hours afterwards, I will invariably gain two lbs. Never one or three, mind you, but always two. It always takes two days for those two pounds to go away, which they will, as long as I stay away from Asian food. Soy sauce is full of both salt and naturally produced MSG, so I have assumed one of them is the cause of this weight fluctuation. I don't have the same response to other salty foods, so it may be the combination of salt and MSG or the MSG alone that are to blame. Whatever it is, it is such a repeatable phenomenon and so easily controlled that I have stopped worrying about it.

Many of the convenience foods people turn to when avoiding carbs are very full of salt, especially cheese, sausages (even healthy ones made with no preservatives) soup broths, salad dressings, etc. All chain restaurant food is full of shocking amounts of salt even though it doesn't taste salty. Many processed foods and almost all chain restaurant foods are full of MSG, too, though it is often hidden in ingredient lists where it might be described as "textured vegetable protein" or even "natural flavoring." Other stealth names for MSG include, "protein isolate," "natural flavors," and "yeast extract."

So if you are having trouble with fluctuating weight when you aren't chowing down on the Pork with Black Bean Sauce check out the labels on what you have been eating to see if you have been boosting your salt and MSG intake without noticing it.

Do I Need to Take a Lot of Supplements When I'm Eating a Ketogenic Diet?

You will only need to supplement if you are eating an extremely low carb diet that has eliminated all grains. In that case, it's a good idea to take a B vitamin supplement, because you might not be getting enough of these important vitamins. If you are eating grains of any kind, this isn't necessary.

If you get dehydrated, potassium might be helpful now and again, but don't take it if you are taking a potassium sparing blood pressure pill. Ask your pharmacist if is safe to supplement with potassium before you try it.

Why Do I Feel like Dead Meat After a Few Months on a Ketogenic Diet?

While some people flourish on a ketogenic diet, others, self included, find that over time their energy levels drop dramatically. This is because of a change in how our thyroid hormones work that only happen to some of us. The technical name for this is "euthyroid syndrome." It isn't dangerous or permanent just unpleasant. It goes away if you raise your carb intake over your ketogenic boundary.

The older I get, the faster that ketogenic diet exhaustion kicks in. If you start feeling that way for more than a week after you've been eating a ketogenic diet for a while, it's time to raise your carbs enough to get your body back to burning glucose as its main fuel. The exhaustion will only get worse if you persist and it can make you depressed. Making yourself stick to a diet when you are feeling increasingly drained makes you more likely to burn out on that diet and may also reprogram the parts of your brain that regulate food intake in a way that makes it all too easy to go on a months-long carbohydrate binge.

How Do I Stop a Ketogenic Diet from Plugging Up My Digestion?

When most people start cutting their carbs they tend to eat more meat and cheese and a lot less fiber than they used to eat. The predictable result is that they quickly get plugged up.

Making yourself eat a couple big servings of healthy low carb veggies every day can help. If it doesn't, a spoonful of Metamucil a day usually resolves the problem.

But Metamucil shouldn't be a long term solution. You really do need to eat your vegetables when you are cutting back on carbs. There are lots of lower carb veggies that will contribute dietary fiber without boosting blood sugar to unacceptable heights. A couple servings of broccoli, cauliflower, brussels sprouts, green beans, olives, mushrooms, romaine lettuce, kale etc. will not only fill you up and contribute nutrients you won't get from pills but will keep your digestive system moving.

Why Does My Pee Smell Funny?

If you cut your carbs to where you are in a ketogenic state you will probably notice a change in how your pee smells. You may also feel irritation around the opening of the urethra. Some of this odd odor may be ketones, which your body eliminates in both your breath and your pee.

However, if you, like many people who cut carbs, are eating too much protein rather than a bit more fat, what you are probably smelling are the ammonia compounds that result from the digestion of that excess protein. Our bodies can't store excess protein. So they use some of the protein we eat to repair our tissues and make new enzymes and hormones. If our dietary intake of carbs is very low, they convert a bit of any extra protein to glucose and then break down what's left so it can be excreted. Since protein is full of nitrogen, our urine ends up full of nitrogen-rich ammonia.

Women may find that this ammonia has a corrosive effect on the tissues around the urethra. If this is the case, cut back on the protein. Too much ammonia in your urine means you are eating way too much protein.

Why Am I Having So Much Trouble Sleeping and Having Weird Dreams?

If you have cut your carb intake down below your ketogenic boundary, your body will be burning ketones for most of its functions for the next few weeks. When this happens people can feel very pleasantly alert during the day and too alert at night. This can make it hard to sleep, and when you do sleep you may have unusually vivid dreams.

This quickly passes. After two or three weeks most of the cells in your body outside of the brain stop burning ketones and switch over to burning free fatty acids. You'll lose that pleasant day time clarity along with the sleeping issues.

Why Is My Spouse Suddenly Pushing All These Carbs on Me?

Two words: Dragon breath.

If you let your carb intake drop to a ketogenic level and eat more protein than you need to supply your actual physical need for protein you will develop bad breath so awful that it will knock flies out of the air should they buzz around your head. It will affect everyone but you, because through some nasty trick of physiology you won't be able to smell it. Breathing into your hand won't help. It will smell fine to you, while becoming an increasingly huge problem for anyone who has to live or work with you.

Unfortunately, because we have a societal taboo about telling other people they smell bad, no one is likely to mention it. I have been approached by quite a few spouses who told me that as much as they supported their spouse's quest for health, the stench they were giving off was more than they could handle.

If you go online and search for explanations you'll find a lot of web pages claiming that what you are smelling is the ketones produced by a ketogenic diet, and that this is normal. You'll also find people advising each other to drink more water and chew breath mints, which won't help.

But the spouse or roommate who starts urging carbs on you has probably read these pages. So after plying you with water and putting breath mints any where you might find them they may start tempting you with carbs in the hope this will take you out of the ketogenic state that has made inhaling the air within three feet of you so intolerable.

It doesn't have to be this way. Ketobreath, as it is often called, is not caused by ketones. It is caused by eating much more protein than your body needs. You can eat a ketogenic diet without giving off fumes as long as you keep your protein level reasonable. This means you will do a lot better eating high fat cheese than you will a 16 ounce steak. Because a safe, healthy, ketogenic diet should be one that is mostly made up of healthy fats, with just enough protein.

You can calculate exactly how much protein you need to maintain your health without turning yourself into a human stink bomb using the nutritional calculator you'll find on my Blood Sugar 101 website.

And if you aren't sure what your stink status is, ask. Given a chance, people who have to live with you will be quite honest if you are failing their personal emissions test.

Why Not Eat a Diet That Is Both Low Carb and Low Fat?

Most people with diabetes do very well on lower carb diets. A few do better on low fat diets, but I have never heard from anyone who didn't deeply regret eating a diet that was both low in carbohydrate and low in fat at the same time.

That kind of diet is a starvation diet. It can do terrible things to your metabolism. It throws it into a panic state where your brain and hormones do everything they can to put some more fat on your bones. You start off losing weight, quite quickly, then weight loss comes to a crashing halt and you start regaining no matter what you eat. If your low fat and low carb diet is extreme enough, it can turn into the kind of all protein diet that unbalances your electrolytes in a way that can kill you.

Several fad diets of this type have swept through the online dieting community over the past decade. One caught on with members of the Low Carb Friends online forum in the early 2000s, after a woman with spectacular before and after weight loss photos showed up selling the plan she claimed had let her lose hundreds of pounds. People lost weight on it very quickly at first, but when the metabolic slowdown hit, it was devastating and resulted in dramatic weight gains. Years later, people who had suffered through this rebound reported that it had taken them years until they could again lose weight on any diet.

The woman with those beautiful before and after photos turned out to be a fraud. The impressive before and after photos weren't photos of her. She was quite obese and ended up in court, sued by the dieters who had paid her a lot of money to join her expensive weight loss club.

But though she is long gone, people pushing a similar ultra low calorie diet, the deceptively named HCG diet, are still at large, though people who have tried that diet have also experienced fast weight loss followed by severe metabolic slowdown and a devastating weight regain. This diet is also a based on a fraudulent concept, as there isn't actually any human chorionic gonadotropin (HCG) in the expensive pills and potions sold by the people profiting from this scam. They get away with this deception because their products are labeled "homeopathic," which is baloney-speak for "there isn't any of the substance named on the label in this bottle."

A moderate carb, moderate fat diet is fine. So is a low carb diet or a low fat diet. It's when you go low on both fat and carb at once that the problems start.

Will Dr. Taylor's Newcastle Diet Cure My Diabetes?

I didn't mention this diet in the previous answer, because it isn't, technically, a scam, but it is yet another extremely low carb, extremely low fat diet. What's different about this one is that it was run under controlled conditions, supervised by a doctor, and its results were published in a major diabetes journal, back in 2011.

At the time, its author, Dr. Roy Taylor, made headlines by claiming to have cured patients of Type 2 Diabetes by putting them on an 800 calorie a day, medically-supervised, low fat starvation diet for six months. In his reports, he introduced some detailed cell studies that purported to give proof that this starvation diet had altered these people's beta cell function in a fundamental way and reduced liver and pancreas fat. But the promised follow-up study that was intended to show how long this cure lasted once people stopped eating that highly restrictive diet was never published.

My guess is that it was because these people's diabetes wasn't cured at all. Their blood sugars improved dramatically while they ate this diet because it was very low in carbohydrate—it's impossible to eat enough carbs to raise most people's blood sugar on an 800 calorie diet. Liver and pancreas fat, if they *did* actually decrease, probably did so because that diet had eliminated the acquired insulin resistance caused by high blood sugars and the high triglycerides that fill the blood when people eat too much carbohydrate. But the diet only lasted six months, which coincidentally is the point where the devastating metabolic slowdown associated with starvation diets kicks in. So it is likely that when people stopped eating his diet they found themselves with disordered metabolisms and brains that were screaming they needed to get busy eating.

If you are tempted to try this approach on your own, *don't*. A diet that low in calories, fat, and carbs can be very dangerous. Dr. Taylor's subjects were fed liquid meal replacements put together by nutritionists who worked out every gram to be sure that they didn't end up with the fatal electrolyte imbalances that are such a threat with high protein starvation diets.

But why be tempted? You can get the same blood sugar improvement eating a diet that provides the same amount of carbohydrate as Dr. Taylor's diet did without requiring that you starve and, most importantly, without putting your body into that devastating famine mode where you end up with a disordered metabolism that makes you prone to binge eating.

Will a Vegan Diet Reverse My Diabetes?

The short answer to this is that a vegan diet will lower your blood sugars to normal levels but only if the vegan diet you eat is one that provides only the amount of carbohydrates you can tolerate. In this regard it is no different than any other diet. The problem with eating a carb-restricted vegan diet is that vegans don't eat any animal products at all. So not only does a vegan diet eliminate the meats, poultry, and fish that you'd cut out on a vegetarian diet, it also forbids you to eat the cheese and eggs that vegetarian low carb dieters depend on to get enough protein.

This isn't to say you can't eat a vegan diet if you feel strongly about avoiding all products associated with animals. But don't expect it to lower your blood sugar unless you also give up most of the grains and beans that most vegans base their diet on. There is nothing magical about eliminating animal products that would make it easier to tolerate the starches and sugars in those grains and beans.

The medical studies the fanatical vegan doctors base their claims on proved that after 74 weeks on a vegan diet, their study subjects had lowered their A1C on average from 8.0% to 7.77%. That is not my idea of "reversing" anything, as that average A1C maps down to an average blood sugar of 177 mg/dl {9.8}. That blood sugar level is high enough to promote all of the classic diabetic complications.

But that kind of outcome is to be expected, as the diets these vegan doctors promote are high carb, low fat diets and those diets have *always* given people with diabetes blood sugars in this range. That is why so many people with diabetes who have followed the traditional low fat/high carb diabetes diets that have been recommended since the late 1940s, have ended up with heart disease and complications.

Once you have eliminated all animal related products it becomes extremely difficult to eat a strict vegan that cuts down on carbs, because the only protein sources left to you are grains, beans, and nuts. The only beans that contain a lot of protein are soybeans. Soy-based foods contain chemicals that damage your gut lining and lead to leaky gut syndrome. That can let plant proteins like gluten leak into your blood stream where they may provoke the antibody attacks that can lead to autoimmune conditions, including Type 1 Diabetes. So a diet high in soy is a very poor choice for anyone.

So that leaves the starchier beans, grains, and nuts as protein sources. You need a lot of beans and grains to get enough protein to avoid muscle wasting. So eating them will raise blood sugars quite high—hence those 7.7% A1Cs the people ended up with in the oft-cited vegan "diabetes reversal" study. Nuts are the other source of useful protein. If you can enjoy eating a diet made up primarily of leafy greens, non sugary fruits, and nuts, go for it, but be careful that you are getting enough protein to avoid muscle wasting. It takes a while for the damage due to eating a diet too low in protein to show up, but over time it damages all your organs, especially your heart.

If you don't want to eat animals for ethical reasons, it's a lot easier to eat a heart healthy, blood sugar friendly, vegetarian diet that still allows you to partake in animal products that don't involve killing any animals. Egg and dairy products easily provide the protein you need to satisfy your appetite and keep your organs healthy, and the variety they provide that will keep you from burning out on your diet after a year.

What About Intermittent Fasting?

After seeing some people I know who had always had a very tough time sticking to diets lose impressive amounts of weight on a 5:2 intermittent fasting diet, I decided to give it a try. There was some research suggesting intermittent fasting might have some useful metabolic benefits, and after so many years of keeping a close eye on calories I couldn't help but be seduced by the "eat all you want and lose weight" results my friends' experiences suggested were possible.

It was a mistake.

Though it wasn't a starvation diet, it ended up acting like one. I experienced seven months of dramatic and easy weight loss, which even got rid of the stubborn subcutaneous fat on my tummy. The diet lowered my blood sugar and my blood pressure. But those first blissful months were followed by several years of complete and utter metabolic slowdown.

My weight loss first stalled. Then the weight came roaring back, as it did for my friends, and nothing we tried would make it stop. My appetite became unmanageable, and all I wanted to do on the days I wasn't fasting was eat. My estrogen levels, which had been steady for a decade, also crashed, and I ended up suddenly developing severe menopausal symptoms. I kept on fasting twice a week, tweaking this and that, but after two full years I admitted defeat. I ended up at the same weight I'd started out with, but with a lot more subcutaneous tummy fat.

While eating the 5:2 diet I participated daily in an online support fasting diet support community. Almost all the participants were women 40 years old or older. A few of us had diabetes, the rest did not. And guess what, almost all the other middle aged women dieters in that support group experienced the exact same result. No matter what they tried, their weight loss stalled and then slowly they started gaining again. Many developed the same problem I did with binge eating. Nothing anyone tried got the diet working for them again. People tried eating strict low carb diets. They counted calories. They tried fasting an extra day each week. It didn't help.

The research upon which all the health claims for intermittent fasting rests was all conducted in small groups of people who were studied for only a very short time. Many of the study subjects were younger males. (The people who are singing the praises of this diet online are all males too.). Since the diet works beautifully for almost everyone for those first six months, these kinds of studies will continue to make it attractive. Until there are much larger, longer studies we can only guess at what they will show. My guess is that they may find that intermittent fasting is a very bad choice for middle aged and older women. I can't say much about what impact it might have on men because there were too few males reporting to the support group to draw any conclusions.

People with diabetes who already have enough trouble with their weight should fight the temptation to try this latest miracle cure until there is some better quality research that tracks the effect of this diet on people who eat it for longer than one year. If it turns out that the problems only affect middle aged women, it might turn out to be safer for younger people and men. But there isn't any long term data to support this conclusion now.

If you can't resist trying one of these diets, don't do it for more than a few months at a time. Then stop and maintain your weight loss without fasting for a few months, to see if you can do it. If while you are actively fasting, you find yourself eating way too much on non-fast days, take a break. It's a sign your body is getting desperate to replace the fat you've lost, and a desperate diabetic body determined to regain body fat is not the body you want to be walking around in.

Why Does Fasting Make My Blood Sugar Go Up?

The same stress hormones that cause dawn phenomenon, which is discussed on Page 123, can make it so that when people with diabetes fast, their blood sugars continue to rise. The only way to stop that rise is usually to have something to eat. So if you do feel you have to try an intermittent fasting diet and see your blood sugars rise, design your diet so that you eat a little something when you get up to stop that morning blood sugar rise continuing.

How Can I Keep From Falling For These Fad Diets?

We all do, once or twice, self included. It would just be so nice if there was a simple, easy way to solve all our diet problems! But to keep you from having to make all the mistakes we grizzled elders have made, here's a checklist to help you determine which writers to trust:

❖ Has the writer trained in a medical specialty where they would actually treat people with diabetes for diabetes? If not, what special knowledge does he base his claims on? Note I'm using the male pronoun here because 99% of the MDs who write bestselling books purporting to cure diabetes with diet are men. The bestselling diet books written by women are written by aging movie stars or personal trainers.

❖ Does this author himself have diabetes? There are only three authors I know of who write about diabetes who themselves have long experience living with diabetes: Dr. Richard K. Bernstein, Gary Scheiner, and Gretchen Becker. Bernstein and Scheiner both have Type 1 Diabetes. Unlike the MDs whose ghostwritten cure-all diet books become bestsellers, these writers with diabetes offer solutions that are complex, explained in great detail, and not something you could compress into a sentence of 25 words or less. People who actually deal with diabetes day to day and year to year have learned that diabetes *is* complicated and that there are no simple solutions. Living a healthy life with diabetes requires hard work, an open mind, and a lot of study.

❖ Has this doctor written other books, and if he has, do they target people with other difficult to manage chronic diseases and offer the same solution to sufferers of each one? It's a huge red flag when a doctor writes the same book promoting the same simplistic solution for people with conditions as different as cancer, dementia, and chronic pain. Each of these conditions is complex and they have in common only that they are often fatal and there are few effective treatments. Quacks gravitate towards patients with these kinds of conditions because they are the ones most desperate for a cure and hence the easiest to exploit.

❖ Does the author claim to be an alternative medical practitioner? This isn't always a huge flashing red light, but the term is one that quacks love to adopt to explain why they have no hospital affiliation or other mainstream medical credential.

❖ Is Dr. Miracle Cure a medical doctor? People with PhDs in any subject, including English Lit, can legally call themselves "Doctor." What they can't do is put the initials MD after their names. Chiropractors also may call themselves "doctor," but only MDs and DOs have graduated medical school.

❖ Does the author's solution require you to adopt an extreme diet? If the book is a huge seller, the answer is almost certainly "yes." Publishers love books along the lines of "The No Red Food on Thursday Diet" or ones that promise you could cure what ails you simply by eliminating all the foods you enjoy eating and replacing them with obscure vegetables hitherto consumed only by natives of an archipelago off the coast of Africa. People are always more enthusiastic about something exotic they've never tried than the things they've tried before that didn't work.

❖ Have you ever run into anyone who has eaten the way the doctor tells people to eat for more than two years? My research into low carb diets and how they compare to other diets, which is described in my book, Diet 101, turned up the fact that no extreme diet of any kind works for more than a year for most people who try it. Few work for more than six months. When people do stick to an extreme diet for six months or more, they are still likely to end up in worse shape two years after starting than they were in when they began due to burnout and to some nasty metabolic effects that occur after people eat extreme diets that lead to binge eating and slowed metabolisms.

❖ If the doctor claims to treat people with diabetes in a clinic, have you ever seen anyone online posting about visiting this doctor? If you did, did they post other messages about topics unrelated to the greatness of this doctor? People who only post about a single cure are often paid shills.

❖ If the doctor cites research, go online and read the study cited. Check that it wasn't published in a vanity journal. (see Page 108). If it was published in a legitimate journal, it still may not prove what the author says it does. Look at the size of the population studied and how long they were studied for. Studies of 10 or 20 people who ate a diet for two weeks tell you zero about how a diet will affect your body over two years. To be meaningful, diet studies need to involve hundreds, if not thousands, of people and last at least a year with follow up a year or two later to track whether people could stick to the diet that long and to see if the benefits that were seen in the early days of the diet persisted. You are going to have diabetes for a very long time, we hope, so you need a diet that keeps working 5, 10, and 20 years or more.

Chapter Five

What Else Will Lower My Blood Sugar?

Are Supplements Safer Than Prescription Drugs?

The supplement industry has worked tirelessly for the past 30 years to convince Americans that completely unregulated, so-called "natural" supplements are safer and more effective than the pharmaceutical drugs your doctor prescribes. This claim is made despite the fact that almost all supplements—and all vitamins—are manufactured in China, where water and air are full of toxic chemicals banned here in the United States and there is a long history of consumer fraud.

Many countries do regulate supplements, but not the United States. Here dietary supplements are, by law, completely unregulated. That means no one checks what is actually in the pill or capsule supplement a company sells unless there are multiple reports of death or very serious side effects linked to a particular company's supplement.

Waving the banner of "Freedom of Choice," the supplement companies have made it legal for them to sell you bottles full of nothing but grass clippings and calcium phosphate. Billions of dollars worth of fraudulently labeled bottles of each are sold each year to trusting consumers who believe they are swallowing valuable exotic herbs and powerful micronutrients. This isn't a guess. Every now and then journalists take bottles of supplements to the lab and get them analyzed. That is often what they find.

Unfortunately, the journalists never tell you which brands turned out to be nothing but grass clippings. Huge, highly profitable supplement companies have enough money to pay for lawsuits that could bankrupt a newspaper or TV channel even if the supplement companies lost.

So though every single supplement company claims to sell nothing that isn't utterly pure, we know for a fact that half of them are lying. Even when companies provide documentation purporting to prove that their wares have been certified by a lab, the fine print reveals that only one batch of the supplement was tested and certified, often years before your bought your pills. There is no ongoing testing taking place.

The supplement business gets a huge boost from websites run by MDs who derive most of their income from selling self-branded supplements rather than practicing medicine. Why spend all your time dealing with sick people and insurance companies when you can slap your own labels on boxes of generic supplements, pay an agency to write a convincing sales spiel for your website, and golf while the earnings pile up. And pile up they do. These doctor-branded supplements may be priced at ten times what they cost the doctor.

The sales pitches these credentialed hucksters use may suggest that mainstream medicine is trying to keep you from knowing about the magical cure the huckster is selling. They often include an incomprehensible but scientific-sounding explanation of why only a very special, left-handed, cross-eyed, or midnight-harvested version of the supplement, available only from the huckster, will be effective. This helps sell product, because customers may have already tried the same supplement in the past and not had good results.

People often do feel much better after paying $50 for a bottle of grass clippings. That's because people often feel better after swallowing *any* pill they have been told is a powerful drug even if it is just plain calcium phosphate or a sugar pill. This is called "the placebo effect." It is so predictable that legitimate drug companies have to compare any new drug they hope to get approved to a pill with nothing in it, just to prove that their drug is actually doing something real.

Researchers have also found that the prices people pay for placebos influence how well they work. People with Parkinson's disease feel a much stronger effect from an injection of water with salt in it when they are told it costs $1,500 than they do when they are told it only costs $100. I suppose this offers some justification for those web-only doctors who sell bottles of nothing for $65 apiece, when you could buy the same bottles of nothing for $6.99 at CVS.

But all this explains why I am wary of supplements, especially the very expensive ones that are pitched to people with chronic illnesses. Over the 19 years that have passed since my own diabetes diagnosis I have seen dozens of these miracle supplements come and go. None has ever lived up to the claims made for it. Some turn out to be harmful.

A very few seem to have some use, but when this is true you will get the same effect from the cheapest drugstore branded version as you do from the $60 bottle some defrocked MD is hawking on www.expensivecures.com.

If you want to know more about the supplements reliable research has found might be useful for people with diabetes, visit the web page "Helpful Supplements for Diabetes," which you'll find at **http://www.bloodsugar101.com/20144672.php** You'll find many of the rest discussed on the page "Worthless or Dangerous Supplements" at **http://www.bloodsugar101.com/15877514.php**. Just remember that you have no guarantee that the useful supplement you paid for is actually in the bottle you purchased. The higher the price of the supplement, the more likely that is to be true.

What About Berberine?

Over the last few years I've been bombarded with people asking me questions about berberine, a Chinese herb that appears to lower blood sugar. Maybe it works. People keep writing to tell me it does, and there is a small possibility that some of them don't work for companies that sell berberine. But because we don't know how it works I stay away from it.

Berberine has long been a part of the traditional Chinese herbal formulary. The problem is that lots of things that have been part of traditional formularies turn out to be very dangerous. Chinese herbalists turn out to suffer from kidney cancer at a rate far higher than the general Chinese population. One reason might be that because of the extreme levels of industrial pollution in China there turns out to be a lot of heavy metals like lead and cadmium in Chinese herbs. They may also be contaminated with pesticides that aren't legal in the United States.

And it gets worse. Some Chinese herbs turn out to be effective because they are contaminated with cheap pharmaceutical drugs. In the case of diabetes drugs, past investigations have found first generation sulfonylurea drugs in herbal preparations that were sold to lower blood sugar. These drugs will indeed lower blood sugar, but they will also raise the risk of having a heart attack. That's why they are no longer prescribed in the United States.

Even if an herb isn't contaminated, you have to wonder how exactly it is lowering your blood sugar. You can lower your blood sugar by damaging your liver so that it can't dump glucose anymore, and several supplements that have gone out of vogue have done just that. But damaged livers eventually stop working and then you die. That's why alcoholism is not recommended as a cure for diabetes. Drinking a bottle of scotch a day will lower your blood sugar quite nicely—until your liver turns into a rock and it's lights out. Vanadyl sulfate is another outmoded cure *du jour* that was dropped because of indications it might be lowering blood sugar by damaging the liver.

Your pharmaceutical drugs, as "unnatural" as they might be, are tested routinely and if they fail their tests, the FDA closes the factory that makes them until the problem is fixed.

But I Found This Study That Says...

One of the biggest scams used to sell you supplements, questionable diets, and every other bogus cure that takes advantage of people with serious chronic illnesses is the publication of studies in 'pay to play" fake medical journals that people who aren't familiar with medical research assume are legitimate. The Internet has made it possible for shysters to publish hundreds of these online-only journals that will publish anything in return for a three or four thousand dollar fee.

And by anything, I mean anything. Back in 2013, a bunch of real scientists put together a fake, scientifically ridiculous study and submitted it to hundreds of these online journals, using the names of imaginary professors at a nonexistent university in an obscure Third World country. More than 150 online journals accepted the paper and offered to publish it for fees that ranged up to $3,100.

Many of these fake journals, not surprisingly, have given themselves names that are confusingly similar to the names of legitimate journals. These pay-to-play journals publish a lot of the research you see cited on the websites of supplement profiteers.

If you are influenced by something you have seen described in a study, check out the quality of a journal in which a study has appeared. To do this, go to Google Search and type in the journal's name followed by the words "impact factor." The impact factor is a measurement of how often the journal's articles are cited in other journals. Impact factor values range from a high above 30 to below 1. Higher is better. Journals with impact factors of 3 or more are usually legit. Those with factors below 1 should be treated with suspicion.

If you have a couple thou to spare and have always wanted to see your name atop a published medical research paper, invent a study that uses made up numbers to prove something along the lines of how a novel terpene extracted from bovine earwax lowers blood sugar. Award yourself an honorary PhD and send your masterpiece off to the *Journal of Human Nutrition and Dietetics* or the *Journal of The American Nutraceutical Association*. Then get out your checkbook.

Will Smoking Marijuana Help or Harm My Blood Sugar?

Unfortunately, the demonization of marijuana by the federal government has made it impossible for anyone to do the kind of research that could answer your question. The few studies we have of marijuana's effects are mostly published in fringe journals. So most of what we know is anecdotal.

People who live in states where marijuana is now legal have learned that there are hundreds of different strains of marijuana, all of which have differing properties. Where diabetes is concerned, the biggest issue is how they affect hunger. As anyone who has been to college — and quite a few high school students — have learned — smoking dope can give you the munchies. That makes it very useful for people undergoing chemotherapy, who lose their appetites and can waste away. But wasting away is not a big problem for most people with Type 2 Diabetes.

But there are strains of marijuana that are cultivated for pain relief that could be very helpful for people with diabetes. These strains typically don't make you feel stoned and most importantly, they don't make you hungry. If you can access some of these pain-relieving strains legally, you may find them very helpful for soothing your painful feet. They can't be any more harmful for you than the barely effective, addictive, pharmaceutical drugs that doctors are currently prescribing for diabetic nerve pain.

There is supposedly no documented case of a person dying from a marijuana overdose. The main hazard of this drug is that it can land you in jail or lose you your job if you are subject to drug testing. But if you live somewhere where marijuana is legal, you can answer the question of whether it does in fact lower blood sugar by trying some out and testing your blood sugar a few hours later to see what happens. It may take a week or so to see the full effect. Just avoid the strains prescribed to people with cancer to increase appetite or cure nausea. And lock the fridge if you aren't sure what the strain you are testing might do.

What Supplements Do You Take?

Like most people diagnosed with Type 2 Diabetes, I bought my share of supplements over the first couple years after my diagnosis. That's how I learned how useless the cures *du jour* that were popular around the time when I was diagnosed were. So yes, hope springs eternal, but eventually we learn.

I have found a very small number of supplements that do seem to be reliably effective when I buy specific brands. But as I keep pointing out, we are all different. So the few supplements I find useful may do nothing for you.

The ones I currently take are:

Fish Oil—I take it not because it has any effect on heart disease—that has been pretty thoroughly debunked—but because it helps keep my aging eyes from drying out when the humidity drops. I buy the enteric coated stuff so I don't keep burping up this awful tasting stuff. I buy whatever brand is cheapest at my local drug store when they have the buy-one-get-one-free specials they run every so often.

Magnesium Oxide—I take it because it has a very positive effect on my blood pressure. I have had very bad reactions to all the prescription blood pressure medications that work well for most other people, so I'm glad to have found something helpful. Though I also find it is more helpful if I give it a break now and then. I have tried all the much more expensive versions of magnesium which are pitched as being far more magical, but only the cheap oxide version I buy at the grocery store does anything for me.

Melatonin—I take melatonin as a sleep aid because I'm at an age where it can be very hard to fall asleep. I'm not sure if it is a placebo or not, but since it works I keep taking it. The Source Naturals sublingual version works best for me. It sends me to sleep but doesn't leave me groggy the next day the way other brands do. Avoid the high dose versions of this stuff as it only takes a very small amount to be effective and high doses may suppress your own melatonin secretion.

Vitamin D2—I take 1000 IU of drug store brand Vitamin D2—the kind that comes in oil capsules—every couple days in the summer when I spend a lot of time out in the sun. I take the same dose daily during our dark New England winters. It makes a real difference in my mood, especially in those long winter days. I don't believe it has any other significant health effects as none of the advantages claimed for it have stood up to rigorous testing.

But I learned the very hard way that taking too much Vitamin D when your levels are normal can lead to a dangerous build up of calcium in your blood. This raises your risk of heart attack because that calcium turns into plaque. In my case, too much vitamin D—prescribed by my endocrinologist—led to high blood calcium levels that over the course of a year pushed up my blood pressure. It has never entirely recovered. It turned out that my blood Vitamin D levels had been fine before I started over-supplementing. If you take more than a very small dose, get your levels checked and don't buy into the idea that high values are better than ones in the lower half of your lab's normal range.

Vitamin B-12 — The drug, metformin, can impair our ability to absorb vitamin B-12, which can cause a form of neuropathy that looks like diabetic neuropathy, but isn't. Neuropathy caused by vitamin B-12 deficiency can't be reversed. So I take a little bit of this vitamin now and then and get my B-12 levels checked every couple years.

That's it.

Can I Control My Blood Sugar with Exercise Alone?

Most doctors will assure you that the most important thing you can do to improve your blood sugar is exercise. I have polled people with diabetes who have achieved and maintained very good control to see how much a role exercise played in that good control. About half of them reported that exercise made a real difference in their blood sugar. The others said that while it had other benefits in terms of fitness and, perhaps, cardiac health, it didn't make a difference in their blood sugar control.

I believe this, since I fall into the category of people who haven't seen exercise make much difference. There have been long periods of time when I couldn't exercise due to severe problems with my spine — I have popped discs all the way down from my neck to my tail — but my control has been the same during those sedentary periods as it is when I am doing 45 minutes of treadmill six days a week at the gym.

Exercising while eating a low carb diet pushes my blood sugar low, which makes me very hungry. This turns out to be a common reaction. Many people who exercise, both those with diabetes and with normal blood sugars, have a tough time controlling their appetites and food intake afterward, especially women.

The only person I ever heard from who was controlling entirely with exercise was someone who was doing several hours a day of intense exercise. This may work for a while, but over-exercising over a long period of time can wreak havoc on your joints. I'm in my late sixties now, and just about everyone I know who used to do 100 mile bike rides, run half marathons, or pump huge amounts of iron is facing knee and/or hip replacements. And these are people with normal blood sugars, not folks with diabetes, whose tendons and disc material may have been made crispy by years of exposure to high blood sugars.

So I'd suggest that if you decide to use exercise to control your blood sugar, you think through what the long term impact of your chosen exercise will be on vulnerable joints. Choose moderate forms of exercise that don't lead to repetitive stress injuries. Walking is probably your best bet, even though it doesn't give you bragging rights when your friends are all training for marathons. But the whole point of getting our blood sugars under control is to make it possible to live on into our 70s, 80s, and 90s. That is only going to be enjoyable if you've taken good care of those joints.

Does Exercise Cure Insulin Resistance?

Another reason I am not as enthusiastic about exercise as your doctor might be is that your doctor has been sold the line that exercise reduces insulin resistance. Since many doctors believe it is insulin resistance that causes your Type 2 Diabetes, it seems like a no brainer that exercise will cure what ails you.

Unfortunately, this idea is not really supported by the research so often cited to advance this claim. What these studies found was that exercise really only "lowered insulin resistance" for an hour or two after the exercise session. Then insulin resistance came right back. Furthermore, the way that "insulin resistance" was measured in these studies was usually by measuring blood sugar levels before and after exercise, not by seeing how much insulin it took to lower blood sugar a set amount—which would have been far more expensive.

So what these studies really showed is that exercise burns off a bit more glucose than usual. This is a fine way to lower your blood sugar after a meal, especially if that meal was full of carbs. But you aren't making any fundamental change in how your cells process glucose. At best you'll have lowered your blood sugar enough to eliminate the acquired insulin resistance we described on Page 40. But that kind of insulin resistance will come right back as soon as you down a "healthy" fruit smoothie after your exercise session is over and push your blood sugar back over 200 mg/dl {11.1}.

Your innate insulin resistance is what it is. Exercise won't change it. I have heard from many people who have used exercise to lower their blood sugar who report that many years of exercising hasn't led to even a gradual improvement in their blood sugars. To be able to make a case that exercise is making some permanent change in insulin resistance you'd have to see a significant, lasting improvement in how much carbohydrate you can tolerate, even on days when you haven't exercised

Will Exercise Cause Weight Loss Without Dieting?

Exercise alone will not cause more than a tiny amount of weight loss, one or two pounds a year, unless you are pursuing high intensity exercise for four or five hours a day.

The numbers supposedly telling you how many calories you have burned that you see on various gym machines are way too overoptimistic. They greatly exaggerate your actual calories burned. It only takes one nut-filled energy bar to replace what most people have burned off during a typical exercise session.

Several other factors lower how effective exercise is in burning off calories. "Training effect" kicks in, which means that the more you perform a particular exercise, the more adapted your muscles become to doing it and the less calories they burn. Middle age also decreases the effect of exercise, particularly for menopausal and post-menopausal women.

The perky young trainers at the gym, who are all far too young to have any idea what it takes to deal with the weight issues so common in middle age, will tell you that exercise builds muscle and that this extra muscle burns more calories. It's an enticing theory and sells a lot of gym memberships. But in the real world, middle aged and older people can't put on enough muscle to burn a significant number of extra calories unless they adopt regimens so aggressive they are likely to damage discs, joints, and tendons.

Why Does My Blood Sugar Go Up Not Down When I Exercise?

Gentle exercise, such as taking a long walk, will get your muscles taking up glucose from the blood stream and burning it for energy. This will result in lower blood sugars. But if you push yourself harder you may find that intense exercise makes your blood sugar rise not drop. This is because strenuous exercise can get the adrenaline flowing, and one effect of adrenaline—a stress hormone—is to raise your blood sugar. This is the famous "fight or flight response.

In a healthy person, this would be useful. If that tiger is chasing you, that extra blood sugar might allow you to put on the burst of speed that saves you from becoming tiger chow. But in the absence of tigers, those stress hormones just push up your blood sugar. Stress hormones also make you more insulin resistant than normal for the hours that follow a physiologically stressful event. This makes it harder to lower your blood sugar.

If you see your blood sugar going up, not down, after exercise, there are two ways to correct it. You can change when you exercise so you don't start your exercise session with a blood sugar that is already pretty high. Alternatively, you can cut back on the intensity of your exercise regimen until you find a level where your blood sugar goes down, not up. Then as you get fitter, you can gradually work up to more intense levels.

Why Am I Hypoing When I Exercise?

Two things can cause unpleasant attacks of low blood sugar in people who have brought their Type 2 diabetic blood sugars down into the normal range. One is metformin. Metformin limits your liver's ability to dump glucose. This is very helpful at mealtimes, because many people with Type 2 Diabetes have livers that keep on dumping glucose even when glucose is coming in from the meal they just ate. But when intense exercise burns through your blood glucose, you *want* your liver to be able dump enough to top it off again.

If you exercise while eating a ketogenic diet you can run into the same problem. That's because when you eat a ketogenic diet you burn through most of the glycogen stored in your liver. This makes your midsection feel skinnier, which may be very satisfying, but when you run out of blood glucose, there isn't that nice emergency glucose store available to your liver.

Neither metformin nor a ketogenic diet completely stops the liver from storing some glucose, so you don't need to panic if you experience an exercise-induced hypo unless you are also using insulin or an insulin stimulating drug. You'll feel shaky for a while, and may be more insulin resistant for a few hours, but you aren't likely to pass out or die.

The way to prevent this kind of mild hypo is to bring some glucose or candies made out of dextrose with you when you do strenuous exercise. Take a few grams of glucose every so often, enough to push your blood sugar up 10 mg/dl {.6}. The exact amount depends on your body size, but should be no more than four or five grams. The table below shows how much glucose it takes to raise a person's blood sugar 10 mg/dl {.6}. As you can see from this table, the amount depends on their body weight.

Your Weight (lbs)	Glucose Needed (g)
140	2
175	2.5
210	3
245	3.5
280	4
315	4.5

If you are injecting insulin or a drug that stimulates insulin secretion, you should always bring along glucose tabs or dextrose candies when you exercise. Stop to measure your blood sugar every 15 minutes or so. Don't wait until you feel shaky to take some glucose, as a hypo with insulin working can come on quickly be a lot scarier than the kinds you have when you aren't using the stuff.

Will Building More Muscle Lower My Blood Sugar?

The standard advice is that the more muscle you have, the more glucose you will burn. But if there is something not quite right in your muscle cells, so they can't burn glucose properly, you can build all the muscle you want but it won't make all that much difference. Many insulin resistant people with Type 2 Diabetes are insulin resistant because there *is* something wrong with their mitochondria, the organelles within the muscle cells that turn glucose and fat into energy. Though a lot of people with Type 2 Diabetes do report that they exercise, I don't hear from people saying that they have found muscle building has had a significant impact on their blood sugar control.

You can always try it, but my impression is that this theory, like so many others, is widely believed because it has been heavily marketed by the people selling muscle building supplements, personal training, and gym memberships,

Help! Every Time I Get Serious About Exercise I End up Hurt

You and everyone else!

We are currently facing an epidemic of gym-created joint and tendon injuries, which is reflected by the surge in joint replacement and back surgeries. Why? Because people have been sold the idea that extreme exercise regimens are healthy, when the truth is that most of them result in repetitive stress injuries that over time erode cartilage and bone.

Human bodies did not evolve to lift hundreds of pounds of weight or to run 26 miles at a clip. People forget that the soldier who ran the first marathon—bringing news of the victory in the battle of the same name home—dropped dead at the end of his run. And this was a trained soldier!

In the past, it was commonly understood that people who did strenuous jobs involving a lot of lifting ended up in sorry shape, which is why for the last several thousand years the wealthy have made other people do their heavy lifting.

So if you are smart you will never let some just-out-of-college self-proclaimed "trainer" at a gym talk you into undertaking a regimen that puts undue stress on your joints or tendons. The healthiest older people I have known, who were able to remain active through their 90s, were those who took brisk walks and swam, not those who did endurance sports and extreme workouts.

Beyond the perils everyone faces with over-exercise, there is the fact that, as I've explained in several previous answers, when your blood sugars have been high for a while one of the things they do is damage your tendons and vertebral discs. These tissues don't have much of a blood supply to start with and when diabetes damages the tiny capillaries that feed them, these tissues start hardening up. This makes them much more likely to tear.

If you have ever had carpal tunnel syndrome or a frozen shoulder, assume your tendons are a bit crispy and avoid the kinds of exercise that puts strain on them.

If you start feeling pain in feet, shoulders, elbows, hips, or lower back, do *not* push through it. Tendon, disc, and cartilage injuries need rest to heal. Stressing them when they have just begun to heal is a great way to extend the healing time from a few weeks to as long as a year. And yes, I learned this the hard way too, as I have learned so much about my diabetes!

Can Cleansing Myself of Toxins Improve My Diabetes?

If by "toxins" you are referring to the things that fashionable "cleanse" diets are supposed to remove from your system, the answer is "no." These faddy cleanses are really just short term, very low calorie starvation diets. Some of the fruit-based ones are high carb starvation diets that will not only deprive you of needed protein but also raise your blood sugar. If your liver is working properly it will remove toxins from your blood stream no matter what you eat.

What Other Lifestyle Changes Will Improve My Diabetes?

If you are a smoker, the most important change you can make right now is to stop smoking. Yes, I know this is hard, but the classic diabetic complications are caused by damage to the small blood vessels that supply nerves and tissue. They are called diabetic complications when it's high blood sugar that damages them. But smoking damages them too, so the combination of high blood sugars and smoking gives you a double whammy when it comes to complications. Smoking also makes it much more likely that you will end up with wounds that won't heal and amputations.

I know it can be very hard to quit—as tough as quitting heroin for people with certain genetic makeups. But there are programs and devices that can help you go through withdrawal successfully. It might take a few tries, but keep at it. If you can't do it alone ask your doctor to help you find a program that might finally make a difference.

Gum disease can also worsen your blood sugar and contribute to heart disease because it seems to lead to systemic inflammation. People with diabetes are likely to have gum disease, too. So if you don't already floss daily, start doing it. And if your dentist tells you that you already have gum disease, ask them to treat it aggressively and follow the treatment plan they give you.

If you can afford it, buy organic foods, especially vegetables, to cut down on your exposure to the pesticides and herbicides that have been shown to damage our metabolisms and increase the incidence of both obesity and diabetes. Yes, it costs more, but isn't your life worth it?

Learning how to cook delicious foods at home from scratch can be extremely helpful. I'm not talking about learning how to make some complicated Tuscan entree you might see demonstrated on a TV cooking show. Just learn how to make some of the easy-to-cook foods you are buying in frozen or processed forms filled with a long lists of frankenfood additives. If you can replace foods like roasts, baked chicken, stews, salad dressings, soups, chili, and barbecue with homemade, made-from-scratch versions, the quality of your nutrition will go way up.

If you can find a copy of *The Joy of Cooking*, you'll find a lot of helpful instructions for beginners in its pages and lots of easy recipes to get you started. If you run into an instruction you don't understand, ask an old lady to help you out—or anyone else who learned to cook back in the 1950s or early 1960s before junk food completely took over the world.

If you are buying processed foods, even ones sold in places that promote themselves as selling healthy food, you can protect your kidneys and heart from further damage by avoiding any products whose labels show that they contain added inorganic phosphates. These chemicals include sodium phosphate, disodium phosphate, calcium phosphate, and several others.

These inorganic phosphates are added to keep fats from separating in dairy products and to keep brown coloring from turning black in sodas. They are often found in brined prepared poultry, like rotisserie chickens and Thanksgiving turkeys. For some reason, these very disturbing additives are completely ignored by people who otherwise obsess about their health. Food in so-called health food stores is full of them. But my alarm is based on compelling research. It turns out that high levels of these phosphates in your blood promote the hardening of blood vessels that leads to both heart disease and kidney failure. Since both are a concern for people with diabetes, the less of this stuff you take in, the better off you will be.

There is no way of knowing how much inorganic phosphate is in any food that includes it in its list of ingredients as there is no legal requirement food manufacturers divulge this information. But scientific studies have found that the more of these phosphate additives you eat, the more phosphate is found in your blood stream and that the more phosphate you have in your blood stream, the higher your risk of heart and kidney disease.

The amount of phosphate that is considered safe for daily intake is around 1000 mg. One study suggests that it's very easy to take in two or three times that much over the course of a day if you eat several prepared foods that contain these phosphate additives. This is a concern as other research has shown that eating just twice the normal amount will raise your blood phosphate levels significantly. Unfortunately, since labels don't tell us how much phosphate is in our food, there is no way to track our actual intake.

Brown sodas also contain phosphoric acid, which is metabolized into inorganic phosphate in our bodies. Research has found that just drinking two brown sodas a day, diet or regular, can double your risk of developing kidney disease. Grab the diet Sprite instead of the Coke and your kidneys will thank you.

The last thing you can do to protect your health when you have diabetes is to go way, way easy on all over-the-counter painkillers. All the non-steroidal anti-inflammatory drugs like ibuprofen and naproxen turn out to be bad for both your heart and your kidneys if you take a lot of them over a long period of time.

Taking over 1,000 acetaminophen pills over the course of your lifetime is also associated with a much higher risk of kidney damage. These drugs not only harm your kidneys, but they also raise your blood pressure over time. Aspirin isn't a whole lot better. It can cause dangerous bleeding, both in your stomach and, more worryingly to us older people, in your brain.

This doesn't mean you can't use these painkillers. There are times when they may be necessary. Just think twice before popping one. Do you really need it? If you do take the very lowest dose that stops your pain. This is often much less than what is in the super strength versions that dominate pharmacy shelves.

Did I Fail If I Couldn't Reach Goal Without Drugs?

Many people get religious about controlling their blood sugars entirely with diet and/or exercise. They can be very vocal about how much better it is to avoid using any pharmaceutical diabetes drugs.

That is the best solution if it works for you, and many people diagnosed with Type 2 Diabetes can do it. But this approach doesn't work for all of us, especially those whose diabetes is caused by the inability to secrete insulin properly. For some of us it is too late to rely on diet and exercise alone, as we have lost too many beta cells before learning how important it is to keep our blood sugars below the level that causes glucose toxicity.

If you fall into either category, using one of the safe diabetes drugs will make it much easier to control your blood sugar, and the easier it is to do this, the less likely you are to burn out.

Diet burnout is very dangerous to your health—more dangerous than the safe drugs that could help you lower your blood sugar without the need for an extreme diet or exercise regimen. That's because when we burn out we often give up on the whole idea of keeping our blood sugars normal.

Burnout poses a special risk to people eating very low carb diets. Research has found that when people with normal blood sugars who had been eating a ketogenic diet for six months to a year went off their diets they ended up eating even more carbs than they'd been eating before they started that low carb diet. They also ended up eating a lot more fat—which is not healthy when that fat is eaten along with a full load of carbohydrates. As a result, these lapsed low carb dieters saw their cholesterol, blood pressure, and other metabolic measurements get worse when they burned out. If this is what happens to people with normal blood sugars, you can imagine what happens to people with diabetes who burn out.

So here is another Simple Truth About Diabetes Diets: **Any successful diet strategy for people with diabetes must not only cut carbs, it must cut carbs in a way that doesn't lead to damaging burnout.** It's far better to adopt a less perfect strategy you can stick to for the next 50 years than to be perfect for three or four years and then give up.

So my advice is this: Try the Test, Test, Test Strategy and see how low you can get your blood sugars. If you can get into the safe zone with diet alone, stick with that technique for as long as you can do it without feeling stressed, obsessed, or deprived. For many people this may be for the rest of their lives.

But if the carb intake level that gives you normal, healthy blood sugars is so low that the only diet that gives you blood sugars anywhere near normal is one that is so restrictive it feels like punishment, consider adding a safe and helpful drug to your daily routine. You will learn more about these drugs in Chapter Eight.

Even with helpful drugs, you will have to cut back some on carbohydrates if you want to preserve your health. There is no drug that will let most of us eat 300 or 400 grams of carbs each day. But a diet that lets us eat 100 to 150 grams of carb a day is usually doable. Eating that amount of carbohydrate makes it possible to eat a wide enough selection of foods and to enjoy enough occasional treats to make the diet sustainable over the many decades people with diabetes want to remain alive.

Chapter Six
What Should I Do About *This*?

Why Do Normal Blood Sugars Make Me Feel So Awful?

If your blood sugar has been high for a while, your brain has slowly raised the level it considers to be normal to a much higher than normal level. Then, when you bring your blood sugar down to a truly normal level, the brain thinks you are dangerously low and releases a bunch of stress hormones whose function is to push your blood sugars back up again. When this happens, you get all the symptoms of a real life-threatening low blood sugar attack, which we call a hypo, except that your blood sugar isn't anywhere near the very low levels that define a real hypo—levels well below 70 mg/dl {3.9}.

This "false hypo" is a well-known phenomenon, and the good news is that if you wait it out, your brain will lower the setpoint at which it freaks out to the level where a freak-out is called for, and you will only feel like you're having a hypo when you actually are.

Because false hypos will push your blood sugar back up and leave you more insulin resistant for hours after they occur, they can become a serious problem if you are lowering your blood sugar from a very high level—like a fasting blood sugar near 300 mg/dl. {16.6}. If you keep having them, it's a better idea to lower your blood sugar in stages, lowering your post-meal numbers by about 50 mg/dl for a week or two, and then by another 50 mg/dl, until you get down near normal.

False hypos will also make you very hungry, as your brain, thinking it is running out of glucose, puts out the emergency "*Eat carbs now!*" alarm that makes you ravenous. The cure for this is not to gobble every carb in sight. Many of us have found that just taking in two to four grams of pure glucose when that raging hunger hits is enough to calm it down.

The simplest way to get that glucose is to keep some candies like SweeTARTS or the little rolls of American Smarties around. They are made out of glucose, which is listed on the label as dextrose. Any candy that contains mostly dextrose or glucose will do. You can use the carbs listed on the label to determine how many pieces will give you that two to four grams of fast glucose you need.

If you take those two to four grams of glucose, do it only once. After that, as long as you're sure your blood sugar isn't actually below 70 mg/dl {3.9}, hang on, eat nothing else, and wait it out. It will pass. Pretty soon the only time you'll feel awful is if your blood sugar rises to the very high levels that used to feel normal back at the time of your diagnosis.

Why Can't I Feel It When My Blood Sugar Is Too High?

The very weird thing about blood sugar is that some of us can feel it when it has shot up real high and others can't. I've always been in the group that can. It gives me a really nasty, poisoned kind of feeling where it almost feels like my veins ache. It takes maybe an hour to pass.

Since quite a few people have told me they couldn't feel it when their blood sugars were really high, I ran a poll years ago on the old diabetes newsgroup where I asked people who were working hard on controlling their blood sugars if they could feel their blood sugars surging. It turned out that only about half of those responding could.

I have never found an explanation for what causes this really nasty feeling. But it may be something that only happens to people with diabetes when they have been keeping their potentially diabetic blood sugars in a more normal range for a while and then eat something full of carbs that pushes their blood sugar up unusually high. It seems to take a spike of 150 mg/dl {8.3} or more for me to feel this effect.

Whatever causes it, it is a unique and very unpleasant feeling, very different from the jittery feeling you get when you are having a hypo, false or real. If you are still able produce enough insulin to knock that high blood sugar down pretty fast, you may also end feeling a false hypo reaction later as that high plummets down to your usual fasting level.

Some people who don't feel extreme blood spikes have said they envy people who do, and they have a point. No matter how delicious a very high carb treat might be, the way I feel as my blood sugar rises that 150 mg/d or more is so awful that the memory of it can keep me from indulging again in that particular treat—at least until enough time has passed to make me forget how bad it feels. But though that keeps me eating in ways that prevent the most damaging kinds of highs, it takes all the fun out the kinds of special treats it would be nice to be able to enjoy on those rare "special days" like a birthday or Valentine's day, where a bit of overindulgence could be forgiven.

This ability to feel strong blood sugar surges fades out you start gradually eating more and more carbs because you have fallen victim to so-called "carb creep." It takes a very big, very infrequent surge to produce that nasty feeling. When you are having more and more highs, you get used to them pretty fast. Back when I was first diagnosed, I was experiencing surges at every meal that pushed my blood sugar up over 250 mg/dl {13.9} but I never felt a thing. I have heard from other people who felt normal when their blood sugar after meals was reaching as high as 400 mg/dl. {22.2}. So it seems like that toxic feeling some of us get when we spike up into the fully diabetic range is a sign that we're doing well with our daily blood sugar control. But not everyone who is in very good control will experience this.

Why Can't I Get My Fasting Blood Sugar to Drop?

This is one of the most frequent questions people email me. Getting stubbornly high fasting blood sugars to drop can be the toughest challenge we face when we have Type 2 Diabetes. Lowering our mealtime blood sugars often causes a dramatic drop in our fasting blood sugars, but no matter how perfect our blood sugars might be both before and after our meals, many of us will find that the blood sugar reading we see first thing in the morning is always much higher than what we aim for.

This is caused by something called "dawn phenomenon." It happens because your body prepares you to greet each new day by secreting a small dose of stress hormones. These are meant to give you a bit of extra energy — i.e. glucose — so you can shake off your torpor and go hunting for some food. This happens to everyone, normal or not. But people with Type 2 can't use that extra glucose very well. Worse, stress hormones also make us temporarily more insulin resistant, which is something that people with Type 2 Diabetes could do without.

People who use insulin often may find that they need to use more insulin at breakfast to cover a set amount of carbohydrate than they do at subsequent meals. This is also because those early morning stress hormones have raised their insulin resistance.

Since we are all more insulin resistant at breakfast it's a good idea to avoid the very carby breakfast foods most of us grew up eating. Some people find that eating a very low carb breakfast as soon as they awaken brings a high fasting blood sugar down, as paradoxical as it sounds.

Some people find that a glass of wine before bed lowers their fasting blood sugar. My own experience when I tried this solution was that it worked for about a week and then the effect faded out. Since drinking before bed has been found to interfere with normal sleeping patterns, it probably isn't a great idea for many of us. If you are drinking a lot of alcohol at other times of the day it is an even worse idea. Alcohol lowers blood sugar by subtly poisoning the liver so that it can't provide the steady stream of glucose you need when you aren't eating. This is why alcoholics are prone to having severe hypos. You only have one liver, and it would be very hard to replace. So you want to avoid doing anything that might hasten its failure.

Some people find that eating a high protein snack before bed also brings down their fasting blood sugars.

But many of us find there is no easy fix for high fasting blood sugars due to dawn phenomenon. Some of us just have to live with it. The good news is that it doesn't appear that the high fasting blood sugars you see first thing in the morning will harm you if your fasting blood sugar is only high when you wake up. If the blood sugars you see before meals throughout the day are more normal, you should be fine. As long as your blood sugar is normal four or five hours after you've last eaten, you can be certain that those early morning highs are caused by the burst of stress hormones that occur right before you wake.

This means your blood sugar has probably been normal through most of the night and only rose in the hour or so before you awoke. When that is the case, the dawn spikes you experience should be no more concerning than a brief post-meal spike that resolves in an hour or two.

If your fasting blood sugar is very high first thing in the morning — well over 140 mg/dl {7.8} and your blood sugars hours after you have last eaten also remain high throughout the day, even when you are eating a carb-restricted diet, ask your doctor if you can start metformin. This safe drug often does a good job lowering fasting blood sugar.

If metformin and a low carb diet don't do the trick, it's a pretty good indication that you would benefit from using a basal insulin. Basal insulins are specially designed, very slow-acting insulins whose job is to lower only your fasting blood sugar. Most family doctors will prescribe one, though you may have to eat very poorly for a month or so before your appointment to push up your A1C to a level high enough to convince the doctor you need help.

If you are already using basal insulin or are taking a pill that can cause hypos, you may experience a high blood sugar upon waking that looks like dawn phenomenon but isn't. This kind of first-thing-in-the-morning high happens after you have had a hypo late at night while you were sleeping. This often happens around 4:00 AM, and may be accompanied by nightmares or by a pounding pulse that wakes you at that early hour. You won't ever see a low blood sugar on your meter when you wake, because by the time a hypo wakes you up your stress hormones will have pushed your blood sugar back up.

If you think a hidden hypo is what is causing high readings first thing in the morning, inform your doctor that you seem to be going too low late at night. Ask if you can lower your insulin dose or perhaps split it into two shots, a larger one in the morning and a smaller one in the evening.

If you were already taking insulin or an insulin-stimulating pill at the time when you started working on lowering your post-meal blood sugars, a sudden rise in your fasting blood sugar after you cut back on your carbs may be the signal that your fasting blood sugar control has started to recover, so you are hypoing on your accustomed insulin dose. If so, you need to talk to your doctor about lowering the dose.

But you may find that family doctors aren't aware that waking with a pounding heart and a high blood sugar can mean you are taking too much basal insulin. Some will even tell you to raise your basal insulin dose if you wake up with a fasting blood sugar that is suddenly too high. But if you raise your dose of basal insulin as instructed and see your fasting blood sugar go up, not down, suspect a hidden hypo. Studies with continual glucose monitors have confirmed that this is often what is happening.

Should I Test My Fasting Blood Sugar Every Day?

Many doctors are still telling people with diabetes to use their valuable test strips to test their fasting blood sugar. As we mentioned earlier, this is because they were trained that people with diabetes don't need to test their blood sugar at home unless they are taking insulin. Because the insulin prescribed to people with Type 2 Diabetes is almost always basal insulin, the kind of insulin that lowers fasting blood sugar, it makes sense to tell patients using it to test their fasting blood sugar. If it is too high or too low, the basal insulin dose should be adjusted.

But unless you are trying to adjust your basal insulin dose, it is a waste of precious test strips to test your fasting blood sugar first thing in the morning more frequently than once every few weeks. Use those few, precious test strips your insurer will pay for to test your post-meal blood sugars. If you bring *them* down, your fasting blood sugars will follow.

My Insurer Won't Pay for Enough Strips What Should I Do?

You will probably need more strips than your insurance plan will cover during the first two or three months of working on lowering your blood sugar as you will need to test after quite a few meals to learn what effect those meals have on your blood sugar. So figure on buying yourself some more strips, ideally discounted ones. The cost of these extra strips is a whole lot less than what you will pay in deductibles if you let your blood sugar deteriorate to where complications turn you into a frequent flyer at your doctors' offices.

There are discounted meters and strips available that are much cheaper than the premium brands many insurers pay for. You can get a cheap Walmart store brand meter and strips for a fairly reasonable price. (Of course, that price would be unreasonable for anything else you might ever purchase that involves the same amount of engineering, but strips have been a rip-off as long as I've had diabetes.)

Do *not* sign up for any monthly strip delivery program. You just want a box now and then, and some of those subscription programs can be tough to cancel. Be wary of companies advertising meters that are supposedly ideal for people on Medicare. The meter you can buy at Walmart is likely to be more accurate.

Be careful, too, about buying name brand strips from resellers on eBay or elsewhere online. Some people find this works out for them, but sellers are so anonymous on eBay or websites hosted who knows who, located who knows where in the world, that you never know what you will get. You may get expired strips or strips that have been damaged by exposure to heat or frost.

There are several brands of generic strips which claim to work with brand name meters which you can buy on Amazon. These vary in quality, too. Some work for a while, and then people report that the new ones they buy are random number generators.

You might get useful answers if you ask members of an online support group where you can purchase cheap test strips. Though keep in mind that there are people in these support groups who pretend to be people with diabetes but are really shills who participate in support groups only to push products they are paid to promote. Companies that sell products also host support groups. So be wary of any product that is repeatedly recommended in a support group whose host will sell you that product.

You should only need extra test strips for the first few months of your efforts to lower your blood sugar, especially if you are careful to note exactly what you ate, how much carbohydrate was in it, and what it did to your blood sugar. Once your blood sugar has flattened out, you will know how much carbohydrate you can tolerate and won't have to test meals you know contain a quantity of carbs you can handle.

I Just Saw a Spike to 190 Mg/dl Am I Screwed?

You're likely to see a lot of spikes that high and much higher over the years to come. Don't panic. As you've read elsewhere in these pages, it takes years of daily exposure to high blood sugars to cause the complications we want to avoid. A spike now and then won't cause permanent harm.

If you know what you ate that caused the spike, just add it to the list of things you probably shouldn't be eating very often. If you can't figure out what caused an unexpected spike, here are a few things that might have been to blame:

❖ Test strips may occasionally produce bad readings for no reason at all. If you expose them to intense heat or freezing, that may make it more likely. Meters get less accurate as they age. Low batteries may also need to be replaced in your meter as they, too, can sometimes cause misleading readings.

❖ Sometimes you'll see a shockingly high reading because you got something on your finger that affected the reading. So if you see a really high reading when you didn't expect to, wash your hands, dry them, and then test again.

❖ Sometimes you'll see higher than expected readings for several days in a row while eating foods that you usually can handle. Sometimes this hints that your body is fighting infection, since blood sugars may rise as the immune system mobilizes.

❖ Another problem that could cause an unexpected high is if you have gotten dehydrated.

❖ Some drugs or hormone preparations can also raise your blood sugar. So if you started a new medication recently check its official Prescribing information's "Side Effects" section to see if "hyperglycemia" is listed. This is the fancy term for high blood sugar.

Help! I Can't Stick to a Diet

Sometimes your problem is that you are trying to eat a diet that is too rigid. If after several tries you find it impossible to stick to a particular diet, ask yourself what changes you would have to make to it to make it more tolerable. Sometimes those changes are less dramatic than you might think they would be.

For example, when I burnt out on eating a strict ketogenic diet, I found I did a lot better if I had an off-plan meal every week where I could eat some of the carby treats I had missed so much when I was being too perfect. Surprisingly, one muffin here or there or a restaurant meal where I let myself eat the bread served with my dinner took the edge off of the diet and made it much easier to eat at a much lower carb intake level the rest of the time.

Try to identify what it was about your failed diet that made it so tough to stick to. Sometimes the problem is that you keep finding yourself in situations where there aren't food options that fit your diet, so when you get hungry you end up eating something you later wish you hadn't.

Try coming up with ideas for food options that fit your diet *before* you get into a situation where you really need something to eat. For example, if you keep one or two vacuum sealed mozzarella string cheese sticks in your purse as an emergency snack, it might get you through a shopping trip without the need for a stop at Dunkin' Donuts. A pack of peanuts you buy at a convenience store is another option for when you are really in a bind. Even a convenience store hotdog with all that salt and additives is still a better choice than a pastry or donut. If you are having trouble figuring out what to eat for lunch at work, visit one of the low carb discussion forums you'll find online and search the forum messages to see how other people have solved their lunch problem.

Cooking for a family can be a challenge, too. But if you making truly healthy low carb meals, there will be plenty of good things for them to eat, too. No one is going to suffer if you cut a ton of carbs out of their meals, especially since your kids may have the same diabetes genes as you do. If they want something else, they can make it for themselves. When you buy snacks, breads, and desserts for them, buy the ones you don't like. Most of all, enlist your family's help. Make it clear to anyone you live with that they need to support you as you work towards lowering your blood sugar because the alternative is to watch you suffer the terrible ravages caused by uncontrolled blood sugars. You have a right to ask for that kind support.

If you can't find a way to change your diet so that you can make it work, ask yourself if the diet is really your problem, or if self-destructive urges that have become linked to food are also playing a part. Food is so essential to our existence, and eating is so interwoven with our first relationship with the mother who fed—or didn't feed—us, that diet can become a battleground on which we struggle with crippling psychological issues that have nothing to do with nutrients or blood sugar control.

Quite a few people have found that early childhood abuse or the experience of having been raped makes them feel that they are only safe when they are enveloped in a huge casing of fat. Only when the trauma that caused that need for safety is skillfully confronted and healed will it be possible for someone with those issues to get their diet in order. Even without a trauma history, many of us do equate food with love, while others have learned to distract themselves from feeling bored by eating.

If you aren't feeling hungry but still find yourself eating things you didn't plan to eat or don't want to eat, or if you feel like you can't control what you know is self-destructive behavior, you may find therapy with a trained, skillful, compassionate therapist very helpful, especially one who has battled these same issues themselves.

Just remind yourself that if your current approach to changing your diet isn't working even after you get your blood sugars to flatten out and aren't driven by obsessive hunger, no magical supplement or exotic food will fix the problem. These are many well-understood issues that cause people to fail at diets. Many will benefit from therapy.

The only approach that is *not* helpful is getting mad at yourself for failing, doing the same thing you did before that failed, failing again, and then getting even angrier at yourself. There is nothing as unhealthy as self-hatred. Find someone who can help you be more merciful and loving to yourself, and get through this!

Help! I Can't Stop Eating Before My Period

The hormone changes that occur the week before women get their periods do make some of us feel like we are starving. Unlike our usual blood sugar-related hunger, this kind of hunger does not go away when we cut our carbs. It is caused by the hormonal changes that take place that time of month.

The only thing you can do when this kind of hunger strikes is have patience. Eating won't make it go away, and if you eat enough to push up your blood sugar, you'll feel even hungrier. Fortunately, most of us will only experience this unpleasant hunger for a day or at most two. While you do, remind yourself that nothing you could eat will make it stop and get busy doing something engrossing to take your mind off it.

This period-related hunger seems to be a bigger problem for women who are in the perimenopausal state. In this case, ask your gynecologist if you should be beginning very low dose hormone replacement. Some of us find this very helpful. Metformin might also be helpful as it seems to lower hormone levels.

Help! I'm Losing Too Much Weight

Though most people with Type 2 Diabetes are delighted by the weight loss they experience when they cut enough carbs to achieve safe and normal blood sugar levels, that same weight loss can pose a problem for slim people diagnosed with Type 2 Diabetes. And yes, they do exist, though you'd never know it from what you see in the media.

Doctors have found that slim people diagnosed with Type 2 Diabetes tend to develop more complications than those who are obese. That's because their blood sugars tend to be much harder to control with diet than those of the more stereotypical, obese person with Type 2. The reason for this is that thin people with Type 2 often have a very limited ability to secrete insulin. They still secrete enough insulin that they can survive without injecting insulin, unlike people with Type 1 Diabetes, but just barely. They may be insulin sensitive, too, so the drugs that address insulin resistance do little or nothing for them. But their very low insulin levels make it tough to put on fat, so unlike most people with Type 2 Diabetes they must work hard to avoid becoming dangerously thin, rather than too fat.

I know, I know, most of you reading this are thinking, "That's a problem I'd like to have!" But it is a real problem for those who have it, as being too thin can be dangerous. I get a small but steady stream of emails from people with BMIs of 18 who can't stop losing weight on the only diet that controls their blood sugar, which is almost always an extremely low carb, ketogenic diet.

This isn't surprising. though ketogenic diets often fail to produce dramatic weight loss, they usually do make it extremely hard to *put on* weight. So if you are a skinny person trying to gain weight at the same time that you are struggling to control your blood sugars, a ketogenic diet may not be the answer. Try raising your carb intake to a level that is about 20 grams above your ketogenic boundary and then eat more fat.

If eating that much carbohydrate makes it impossible to keep your blood sugars in the safe zone or if you are still finding it impossible to stop losing weight, you may not be able to control your blood sugar with diet alone. In that case, I would suggest letting your blood sugar rise high enough over a period of about six weeks to produce an A1C that will convince a doctor that you do, in fact, have a problem controlling your blood sugars. Then ask for a prescription for repaglinide.

Repaglinide is an inexpensive generic drug that few family doctors seem to be aware of. You take it before a meal and it stimulates insulin secretion over the next three or so hours. Like all drugs that stimulate insulin secretion, over time it causes some weight gain. Repaglinide may allow you to eat a lot more carbohydrate at each meal while still maintaining healthy blood sugar levels. Start out with a very low dose, as some thin people diagnosed with Type 2 Diabetes have a genetic condition that makes them extremely responsive to repaglinide. A starting dose of 1/4 of the lowest doses tablet would be a good place to start. Only raise the dose if you don't see a response.

If repaglinide doesn't help, take the steps necessary to convince your doctor you need insulin, as you probably do. Lack of insulin may have something to do with why you are so thin.

Must I Stop My Low Carb Diet Because My Cholesterol Went Up?

It is normal for total cholesterol to rise during the first couple of months of a low carbohydrate diet. However, this is often due to rising HDL (the good cholesterol.) Your triglycerides, which are the fraction of your total cholesterol most closely associated with heart disease, should drop when you cut your carbs. The ratio of your LDL to HDL should drop as well, as should your Total Cholesterol/HDL ratio. These ratios are the only factors derived from cholesterol test results that the venerable Framingham Heart Study has identified as being at all predictive of heart attack risk.

Most people find that the longer they control their blood sugar with diet, the better their cholesterol test results will be. Some find that they no longer need statin drugs they've been taking. But be cautious if you are currently taking statins. Don't stop taking them because you've read that a low carb diet is all you need to ensure your cardiovascular health.

If you have had high blood sugars for years, the chances are that your arteries are harder than normal and that they have developed dangerous plaques which may have become inflamed. Statin drugs appear to fight this inflammation, which it is thought plays a part in causing arterial plaques to rupture, which leads to strokes and heart attacks.

So it would not be wise to stop taking statins until you have several years of excellent control under your belt. Even then, it would be a good idea to get yourself thoroughly checked out by a cardiologist before you draw any conclusions about whether or not you should be taking them.

If your LDL remains high, it's worth asking your doctor to order a test that measures the size of your LDL particles. The smaller they are, the more likely they are to form dangerous plaques. Conversely, if you have unusually large LDL molecules, you are much less likely than most people to develop those dangerous plaques. As long as your high LDL is due to very large LDL molecules, high LDL should not be a cause for concern. But if you have a lot of small LDL molecules, you should take the medications your cardiologist suggests.

Why Is My Blood Pressure Going Up, Not Down Now That I've Cut Down on Carbs?

People with diabetes need to control their blood pressure as much as they do their blood sugar. For many people, lowering their carb intake improves their blood sugar too, But it doesn't always do this. It didn't for me.

One reason our blood pressure might go up when we start working on improving our blood sugar could be that we end up eating way more salt when we cut our carbs. So many of the low carb foods that are easiest to grab when you're hungry are salty, like cheese, sausages, bacon, and nuts to name just a few.

If lowering your salt intake doesn't improve matters, another possibility might be that your diet actually is lowering your blood pressure, but it is doing such a good job of it that you are experiencing a rebound high caused by stress hormones that kick in to keep your blood pressure from dropping too low. This might happen if you aren't drinking enough fluids and have become dehydrated. This is more likely to happen when you are eating a ketogenic diet as they can be very dehydrating. When I was having a serious problem with my blood pressure back when I first started a low carb diet testing showed that I was, in fact, dehydrated. Drink more plain water for a few weeks and see if that helps. If it doesn't, boost your carbs well over the ketogenic boundary and see if your blood pressure improves.

Your blood pressure may also go up when you take a diabetes medication that causes your body to secrete more insulin. Higher levels of insulin than you are used to can affect your sodium/potassium balance in ways that make blood pressure rise. Both the older insulin-stimulating drugs like glyburide and the incretin drugs like Januvia and Victoza can do this.

Whatever the cause, if you can't fix this on your own, talk to your doctor about taking one of the blood pressure pills that are safe for people with diabetes. The ones that are *not* safe are any that contain the diuretic, hydrochlorothiazide (HCTZ), as they raise your blood sugar, and the beta blockers, which not only raise your blood sugar but can also turn off hypo awareness. This makes them very dangerous for anyone who uses a drug that stimulates insulin secretion or who is injecting actual insulin.

I Had a Heart Attack Was this Because I Was Eating a Low Carb Diet?

There no credible evidence that eating a diet that provides more than 1200 calories a day and lowers your blood sugar by limiting your intake of carbohydrates will give you a heart attack. You can feel confident that such a diet is safe because that kind of low carb diet has been subjected to some 20 years of hostile scrutiny. The fat-phobic medical establishment ran study after study because they were convinced such studies would document how harmful the diet would be.

They didn't. These diet studies, which I explored in depth in my book *Diet 101*, confirmed that low carb diets are safe and effective. They do not produce more heart attacks or any other negative health outcome than any other diet, be it an extreme Ornish-style low fat diet, a traditional Weight Watchers diet, or the Zone Diet.

The sole documented report of someone who it is believed died because of eating a low carb diet, turns out to be a case of a person who was eating a diet extremely low in carbohydrates and *calories*. Extremely low calorie diets of any type are dangerous. Any diet that requires you to eat less than 800 calories a day for more than two days in a row should only be undertaken under the supervision of a competent nutritionist. That's because these very low calorie diets—and this includes some poorly designed fasting diets—can mess up your electrolyte balance. Electrolytes include sodium, potassium, calcium, and magnesium. When they go out of balance it means that you have way too much of one and way too little of another. If you really mess up your electrolyte balance, your heart stops beating.

Militant vegans, who hate the low carb diet because people eating it eat a lot of meat, poultry, fish, eggs, and dairy, love to point out that Dr. Atkins, who co-opted the ketogenic diet by renaming it the Atkins diet, died of a heart attack. PCRM, the extremist vegan organization headed by Neal Barnard, went so far as to steal the medical examiner's report describing Atkins' corpse and publish it, which was a criminal act. But Atkins actually died of sudden cardiac arrest, which is caused by problems with heart rhythm, not clogged arteries. More importantly, a published biography of Dr. Atkins makes it clear that Dr. Atkins, who started each day out with a big glass of orange juice, was not actually eating the diet that made him such a wealthy man.

So no, eating a low carb diet won't give you a heart attack. But what might is the damage your cardiovascular system accumulated over the many years *before* you started eating that low carb diet. Especially if the diet you were eating through all those many years was full of blood sugar-raising carbs, artery-clogging trans fat, plaque-building phosphate additives, and hormone-unbalancing plastics, plasticizers, pesticides and herbicides.

No diet is going to immediately undo the damage wreaked by decades of eating additive laden junk foods. Since we know that blood sugars rising as low as 155 mg/dl {8.6} one hour after eating are enough to start the process that leads to hardened arteries, chances are that your cardiovascular system is not going to be in tip-top shape when you begin to work on improving your blood sugar.

But that said, the studies intended to show that low carb diets worsened the markers doctors use to evaluate heart attack risk, found, instead that they improved them. The only time the diet was bad for people's cardiovascular health was when they stopped eating a low carb diet but kept on eating the extra fats that are not healthy when combined with a moderate amount of carbohydrate.

So keep in mind the golden rule of low carb dieting: **The more carbs you eat, the less fat you should consume.** If you are eating over 130 grams of carbohydrate a day, ditch the blue cheese dressing.

What Tests Should My Doctor Order?

Most family doctors will diagnose you based entirely on one of two tests, the fasting blood glucose test or the A1C test. If your blood sugars are high enough at diagnosis, they will prescribe you some pills based on the results of these screening tests without doing any further testing to determine what exactly is raising your blood sugar.

Once you are diagnosed, your doctor will almost certainly order cholesterol tests, because doctors believe that all people with diabetes must have heart disease. The cholesterol test also gives them the excuse to prescribe the statin drug they have been brainwashed to believe is all that stands between all people with diabetes and instant death.

A competent doctor should also run a blood test to see how your kidneys are faring. This test will report your creatinine levels and creatinine clearance rate. However, this is a fairly crude test of kidney function and only reports abnormal results when your kidneys have suffered significant damage.

So good doctors will also give you a urine test called the microalbumin test. This test looks to see if your kidneys are leaking tiny bits of protein, which would be a sign that you already have early diabetic kidney disease. You should have one of these tests as soon as you are diagnosed. If it is at all abnormal, you should have a follow up every year to make sure that your kidneys are not deteriorating.

Take an abnormal microalbumin test as seriously as you would the news that your local nuke plant was melting down. Put all your energy into doing whatever it takes to bring your blood sugars down to at least near-normal levels.

Your doctor should also refer you to an ophthalmologist for an examination of your retinas. This requires that your eyes be dilated with those annoying drops that leave you unable to see for hours after the appointment.

If you have crummy insurance or no insurance at all, these tests can be very expensive. If your A1C at diagnosis isn't above 7.5% and you are willing to work hard on your diet, you can put off the cholesterol test and the microalbumin test for another year, when it is to be hoped you will have got yourself some better health coverage.

You can get your retinas checked by an optometrist very cheaply. They will tell you if they see something that would make it necessary to visit an expensive specialist. Optometrists are the eye doctors who have an OD degree, not an MD. They often have offices in the shops that sell eyeglasses. Don't confuse optometrists with the far less trained opticians who make and fit glasses.

If an optometrist tells you that something they see in your retina means you need to see an ophthalmologist, you need to see one. An ophthalmologist is an MD who specializes in the eye, who has been through many more years of training than the optometrist. Ophthalmologists are qualified to do surgery should it be necessary. Visible changes in your retina require an ophthalmologist's care to ensure that you never have to deal with diabetic blindness.

If you see an ophthalmologist who tells you that you have early diabetic retinal changes, and if your insurance will cover it, ask to have retinal photographs taken to document the extent of those changes so that if you see a different doctor in the future they will be able to tell if your eyes are stable or deteriorating.

Most of all, don't let your fear of what might be going on in your eyes keep you from getting an exam. Early changes can be healed up.

Letting denial make you delay diagnosis can result in the very outcome you fear.

Why Is My A1C 4.9% When My Fasting Blood Sugar Is 175?

As explained earlier, the A1C test doesn't actually measure your blood sugar. It measures how much glucose has become permanently bonded to the hemoglobin in your red blood cells. If your red blood cells are normal and live exactly the three months the average blood cell lives, the amount of glucose bonded to those red blood cells can be used to estimate what your average blood sugar has been over the past three months.

Problems arise when your red blood cells aren't normal or don't live the usual lifespan of a typical red blood cell. If you have misshapen red blood cells or red blood cells that die faster than normal your blood cells won't bond with as much glucose. This will give you a normal or low A1C test result, no matter how high your actual blood sugars have been.

Since some doctors are not aware that abnormal red blood cells can render an A1C test result worthless, I have heard of patients who were told they were doing extremely well because their A1Cs were so low, when in fact, they were running blood sugars all day long that were high enough to cause all the diabetic complications pretty quickly.

If your A1C barely reaches 5.0%, but you are seeing very high fasting blood sugars or frequent blood sugars as high as 300 mg/dl {16.6} when you test at home, ask your doctor whether you are anemic. Anemia is frequently the explanation for this kind of discrepancy. If you are anemic, make sure your doctor knows that your A1C test result will not reflect your blood sugars. Bring your blood sugar log with you to your appointment and insist your doctor take a look at those highs.

If your A1C test result is obviously inaccurate, in the future your doctor should order a fructosamine test, instead. That test will be able to track how your blood sugar has behaved over the previous month. If that isn't possible, the doctor should continue to monitor your home blood sugar testing logs and prescribe you more strips.

If My A1C Is Higher Than My Meter Readings Does This Mean I'll Get a Heart Attack?

I often hear from people whose A1C is always higher than expected, who fear this means their risk for heart disease is also higher, given that research has shown that heart attack risk rises step-by-step along with A1c.

But these findings only apply to averages taken from studying very large groups of people. So all it tells us is that a totally average person whose average A1C result, achieved with red blood cells that live an average length of time, develop heart disease in greater numbers when that average A1C rises over 6.0%. There is no data to suggest that a higher percentage of the hemoglobin A1C protein in your blood is what actually causes heart disease.

Until there is some actual research about what happens to people who keep their blood sugars in the normal range but have higher than predicted A1C test results, I think it is safe to conclude that you'll be fine as long as your blood sugars are staying under the post-meal levels that would start or promote the blood-sugar-related processes that harden your arteries.

Some research also suggests that when blood sugars are normal or near normal red blood cells may live longer than average. This leaves more time for glucose to bond to their hemoglobin, which in turn leads to an A1C that is higher than what would be predicted based on what you see when you test your blood sugars at home. This may explain why so many of us in the 5% club have higher than expected A1Cs.

When Should I Go to the ER with A Very High Blood Sugar?

A blood sugar over 500 mg/dl may very well be an emergency, especially if you don't feel well. If you see one when you test, wash your hands in case you got something sugary on them, test your blood sugar again, and if you still see a reading that high, call your doctor's office and talk to the nurse. If they tell you to go to the ER, go. If you don't have a doctor to call, go to an urgent care clinic or if there isn't one available, the ER.

A blood sugar that high is an emergency not because those very high blood sugars will lead to complications. It takes more than a few days of exposure to high blood sugars to do that. It's an emergency because there are two different disorders that can occur when your blood sugar is very high that can kill you within hours.

One is diabetic ketoacidosis (DKA). This is a condition that usually occurs in people who are not making any insulin at all, which usually this means someone with a diagnosis of Type 1 Diabetes. But it can also diagnosed in people with Type 2 diagnoses, because many people who develop diabetes late in life are misdiagnosed with Type 2 when they really have a form of autoimmune diabetes that is killing off all their beta cells.

There is also a brand new reason why people who do have classic Type 2 Diabetes may develop DKA. It turns out the often prescribed new drugs, Invokana, Jardiance, and Farxiga can cause it. This is a recently discovered side effect and many family doctors may not be aware of it.

DKA can be fatal, so don't mess around if you have any symptoms of it. Those symptoms are high blood sugars, meaning blood sugars over 300 mg/dl {16.6} that occur along with excessive thirst, frequent urination, nausea and vomiting, abdominal pain, loss of appetite, weakness or fatigue, shortness of breath, fruity-scented breath, and confusion. If you have strips that measure ketones handy, they will show a lot of ketones. But though you may have heard that spilling ketones is completely normal when you are eating a ketogenic diet, this is only true if you are spilling ketones while running normal blood sugars—and not taking one of these new oral drugs. The combination of high ketones and high blood sugars can be deadly. The new drugs may even cause DKA at much lower blood sugars, which is why for now if you must take one of these drugs you should not eat a ketogenic diet.

DKA is an emergency, but if you get to a hospital when you develop DKA you can be rescued with intravenous insulin and fluids.

The other dangerous condition associated with very high blood sugars that occurs in people with classic Type 2 Diabetes is called the hyperosmolar hyperglycemic state (HHS). Untreated this condition leads to coma and death. It happens when people with Type 2 Diabetes become severely dehydrated at the same time that they are experiencing very high blood sugars. This can happen when they have serious diarrhea and vomiting, as happens when they catch a norovirus, E. coli, or salmonella infection. It also happens to elderly people who are prone to dehydration. With HHS, you won't be spilling ketones. But if it occurs it is more likely to be fatal than DKA. Estimates of its fatality range from 10-20%.

Unlike DKA which develops suddenly, HHS may develop over a course of days or weeks. Symptoms include very high blood sugars, over 600 mg/dl {33.3}, drowsiness and lethargy, delirium, coma, seizures, visual changes or disturbances, one sided paralysis, and sensory deficits. Patients with HHS do not typically report abdominal pain, which is often seen in DKA.

What these conditions have in common is that if you develop them, you can go from fine to dead very quickly, though they can be treated successfully at the ER.

Not everyone whose blood sugar goes over 500 mg/dl develops either condition. And if you have been diagnosed with Type 2 Diabetes and see occasional readings between 300 and 400 mg/dl {16.6 and 33.3}, which most people will, they aren't likely to kill you. Nor does one very high reading mean you have to head for the emergency room if you have access to insulin or a drug you know will lower your blood sugar within an hour or two.

If you use insulin and your high blood occurred because you forgot to take your usual dose or because your insulin spoiled due to exposure to high temperatures, all you may need is another dose of insulin, possibly one from a new pen or vial.

But if your blood sugar does not come down swiftly in response to what you usually use to lower it, or if your blood sugar is over 300 mg/dl and you are vomiting and cannot keep down liquids, or are having a lot of diarrhea, you do need to head to the ER.

If you were only recently diagnosed with diabetes and your meter is reading "HI" or in the 500s and you don't feel well, you most certainly need to head to the ER, because you may actually have Type 1 and have been misdiagnosed.

If you do go to the ER, it's possible you'll end up being told your high blood sugar isn't a crisis and be sent home with nothing more than a huge bill. This may make you think your trip to the ER was a mistake, but it wasn't. Until a doctor examines you and confirms that you do not have DKA or HHS there is no way of knowing whether you have one of these potentially fatal conditions. It's much better to guess wrong and end up with an ER bill than to guess wrong and end up dead.

Why Are Hypos So Dangerous?

We all start out having a built in system that keeps our blood sugar from dropping low enough it could kill us. How this works is that as soon as your brain senses that your blood sugar might be heading for a dangerous hypo it sends out hormones that cause you to get a big burst of stress hormones that will push your blood sugar up again. This is called a "counterregulatory" response. We've already talked about this kind of response when we talked about false hypos, which happen when the brain erroneously thinks a hypo is threatening when it isn't.

But when it is, you want this burst of stress hormones, the more the better. Among other things they cause another pancreatic hormone, glucagon, to be secreted, whose job is to make your liver dump all the glucose it has handy into your bloodstream. When this happens, you'll feel a bit edgy, your heart will pound, and for the next couple hours you might feel more stressed than usual, but that's pretty much it. It's unpleasant, but it won't kill you.

Unless you start hypoing a lot. When this happens, your body gets used to being at a lower blood sugar level, and the threshold where your brain sounds the alarm drops. Blood sugar levels that should trigger a counterregulatory response no longer do. This is described as "losing hypo awareness." When it happens, you can drop into the 50s {2.8} or even lower without even noticing it. This is a problem, because the next step may be that you drop into the 30s or 20s {1.7 or 1.1} without noticing it. When that happens, the crucial brain cells that can't live without glucose will start shutting down.

When you have lost hypo awareness, the only symptom you may have when your blood sugar is dangerously low is some weird visual effects. These seem to start happening when your blood sugar is around 40 mg/dl {2.2}. Part of your field of vision might get all wavy. Or you might lose a chunk of your visual field all of a sudden. This is a major warning sign, because if you don't bring your blood sugar up from that level the next thing that happens is that you become very irrational, can't think straight, and may become combative, just as if you were very drunk. Or you may just pass out. If your blood sugars keep dropping and get close to zero you can die if not immediately treated with a glucagon injection. This is something ambulance crews carry and that people using intensive insulin regimens for Type 1 usually keep handy.

People with Type 2 Diabetes become more prone to hypos when they use insulin or insulin stimulating drugs, especially when they are elderly. This is one reason that doctors under-treat elderly people with diabetes. The combination of a weak counterregulatory response, iffy digestion, and the decline in memory that often occurs as we age makes it too easy for the elderly to hypo. So when doctors do prescribe insulin for people with advanced Type 2 who are over 65, they tend to give them a much smaller dose than the one that, if they were younger, would provide better blood sugar control. This is done as a protective measure, because hypos in the elderly have been found to damage their brains.

When Do I Need to See an Endocrinologist?

You need to see an endocrinologist if the kind of diet we describe in this book, along with metformin and possibly a basal insulin like Lantus, Levemir, Tresiba, or Basaglar, are not giving you blood sugars low enough to prevent complications or if your blood sugars are rising swiftly despite your best efforts.

If you don't match this description, there is no reason to see an endo unless you want a prescription for fast-acting mealtime insulin. To get that prescription, you'll have to be able to document very high post-meal blood sugars. Otherwise an endo visit is only likely to result in a prescription for an expensive and possibly dangerous expensive new pill, or no help at all.

My own experience and that of many people I have heard from is that endos are likely to shoo you out of the office as a time waster unless your A1C is 8.0% or higher.

My 85 Year Old Mother Was Just Diagnosed What Should She Be Doing?

Conscientious children and care-givers who are well informed about diabetes and want to do what's best for an elderly person diagnosed with diabetes often assume that the elder should be using the same treatments that would be best for someone decades younger. But diabetes in frail people 80 years old or older is different from diabetes in someone middle aged and otherwise healthy. So if you are responsible for the care of an elder in their last decade of life, there are good reasons for not going overboard and forcing them to make demanding dietary changes or take powerful medications.

The advice in this book is addressed to an audience whose goal is to avoid developing the terrible complications of diabetes that will emerge starting about a decade after diagnosis and get worse with each subsequent decade. When you have 30 or 40 years ahead of you, the lower your blood sugar is, the better off you'll be. But as people age, other factors come into play.

People in their 70s and older may have other conditions which affect their ability to metabolize the food they eat. People in their 80s may have suffered deterioration in their ability to taste and smell or changes in their digestions that make wasting syndromes a more immediate threat to their health than diabetes. A low carb diet which triggers weight loss in someone already suffering from wasting could be disastrous.

Elderly organs often don't work well anymore, either. So drugs that are safe for younger people may be dangerous for older people whose kidneys and livers no longer filter chemicals from their blood properly. A drug that is safe for most people may build up to dangerous concentrations in an elder's blood if their liver no longer makes the enzymes needed to dispose of it or if their kidneys can't remove it from the blood stream.

Even if these organs are still working, elderly people may have to take a cocktail of drugs prescribed for other conditions unrelated to their diabetes. These can keep the liver from disposing of otherwise safe diabetes drugs.

Problems with balance and blood flow also make many elderly people more prone to fall, which can cause bone fractures that dramatically shorten their lives. Low blood sugars that would be a mild annoyance in a younger, healthier person are much more dangerous to elders because they can cause the dizziness or weakness that leads to falling.

Memory problems, even mild ones, also pose a threat. A failing memory may make it impossible for an elderly person to keep track what they are eating or remember when to take a medication. Older people frequently take too much of a medication because they forget they already took their daily dose. With insulin stimulating drugs or insulin itself, this kind of forgetfulness can be fatal if a person is on an aggressive drug regimen meant to provide normal blood sugars. Even with proper dosing, studies suggest that, unlike people with Type 1 Diabetes who have been taking insulin most of their lives, elders who first start taking insulin late in life are much more likely to suffer severe hypos that send them to the hospital and cause permanent brain damage.

All this should explain why your family doctor may be giving your elderly friend or relative what looks like criminally minimal care. It also explains why some practice guidelines now suggest that people as young as 65 no longer need to achieve even the mediocre 7.0% A1Cs doctors recommend for everyone else. I recently saw an 8.0% A1C suggested as an appropriate target for people over 65 and an 8.5% A1C suggested for those with a limited life expectancy.

But obviously, there is a huge range of health conditions to be found in the population of people over 65. Plenty remain active and healthy into their 80s and might live to be 100 with aggressive care. So a good doctor should be looking at the physiological age of a patient, not their calendar age.

At almost 69 I'm not dead yet. My joints hurt, and my energy isn't what it used to be, but my liver and kidneys are still hauling. I continue to do what I can to keep my A1C in the 5% range. But that said, I am, indeed, more prone to hypos than I was a decade ago, and I am no longer being quite as aggressive about lowering my blood sugar as a result. I also don't diet like I used to because there is quite a bit of data pointing to the conclusion that weight loss for any reason including intentional dieting increases the likelihood of dying in people over the age of 70.

So if an elderly person you care about has been given a recent diagnosis of diabetes and is in decent shape with a mind that appears to be working as well as usual, go ahead, share with them what you've learned about diabetes, then let it go. But be careful not to talk them into believing their doctor is an idiot whose advice they should ignore. You don't know what other diagnoses they have or what other drugs they are taking. Their doctor may have very good reasons for allowing their blood sugar to remain at levels that wouldn't be healthy for you.

Be careful too, about giving advice to an elder who has had poorly controlled diabetes for decades and is now suffering the consequences. It may be too late to reverse the damage. Heart and kidney disease past a certain point in a frail elderly person can't be reversed with diet. You will only add to their suffering if you inform someone dealing with terminal heart disease, dialysis, blindness, or amputations that all that their suffering could have been prevented had they not been the victim of decades of tragically flawed medical advice.

If the elder you are trying to help is your parent, don't expect them to take your advice. When they ignore you, let it go. The more you nag, the more likely they are to refuse to do anything you suggest. That's just human nature. Parents can never quite stop seeing their kids as toddlers. It's hard to take advice from someone whose diapers you changed,

If the older person is no longer able to take care of themselves and you are legally responsible for their care, you may be able to impose a diet or drug regimen on them. But even if the diet you want to impose is a safe and healthy one, you have to put yourself in the elder's shoes and ask whether the benefit the diet or drug provides will make enough of a difference in their quality of their life to be justified.

A person who is 85 years old, mildly demented, and who has other incurable medical conditions isn't likely to live long enough to experience the long term complications of recently diagnosed diabetes. Even if their diabetes is decades old and has contributed to their current, mildly demented, incurable state, it may be kinder to let them enjoy the cake and ice cream which might be the highlight of their day, rather than enforce a strict diet that comes way too late to undo those decades' worth of damage.

The elderly person who is forced to eat a supposedly "healthy" diet may end up feeling deprived or even punished when their favorite foods are taken away. Unless the person themselves is capable of understanding the reasons for dietary changes and has consciously chosen to undertake them, forcing these changes on them may be cruel, not helpful.

My dad ate a very strict low carb diet from his late 30s until his late 90s. After he had the stroke that left him crippled and led to his death a few months later, he ate cookies all day long. I had never seen him eat cookies before, as he was far more fanatical about his diet than I have ever been about mine. But when he knew it was all over, he enjoyed those cookies. When I get to that point I'm going to enjoy my cookies, too. And woe betide anyone who tries to stop me.

Why Does My Family Think I'm a Hypochondriac?

One of the ironies of diabetes is that people will only believe you have it if you take such poor care of yourself that you develop visible complications. Go on dialysis or lose a toe, and everyone will start sending you loving gifts of sugar-free candy.

But if you work your butt off to keep your blood sugar normal, lose weight the way most people do when they cut their carbs, and pass on the chocolate cupcakes with the explanation that you have to keep your carbs down, you are more likely to provoke negative responses. People will warn you that you are killing yourself eating cheese omelets or loudly express disbelief that you really have diabetes since you don't *look* like you have diabetes.

Back when I was using fast-acting insulin to cover my meals, several of my relatives insinuated that my diabetes was all in my head. Another elderly relative responded to the news that I had diabetes by sending me some sugar-packed brownies as a gift. When asked why, they explained it was impossible I could really have diabetes as our family didn't get diseases like that!

So what's going on here?

A lot of times the problem stems from the way that the media reinforces the idea that people with Type 2 Diabetes are lazy gluttons so obese the fire department has to break through their walls to get them to the hospital. If you have worked on your diet enough to have normalized your blood sugar, chances are you are the same size as most other middle aged people. Not slim perhaps, but not likely to be featured on The Biggest Loser. Ergo, you don't look diabetic.

There is also the shame issue involved, especially with relatives. This is also due to the way the media portray diabetes. The tone of voice in which my elderly relative announced that our family didn't get diabetes, was the same one they would have used to explain that we didn't get syphilis.

Even those who support our quest for good health and acknowledge that we do indeed have diabetes may be very resistant when we insist that controlling our diabetes means making significant changes to our diet. They may fear that we have developed OCD as we seem obsessed with counting all our carbs. The blame for this goes squarely on the American Diabetes Association, which has actively promoted the idea that people with diabetes can eat everything people without it eat.

This organization has counted among its sponsors over the years the companies that make sugary breakfast cereals, baked goods, and junk food. "Sponsor" here means "big contributor." So it makes sense that they would promote the idea that you shouldn't stop eating their generous sponsors' products. It also makes sense that the insulin and oral drugmakers, who are the other heavy sponsors of the ADA would also want to publicize this concept, because most people with Type 2 Diabetes who stop eating like everyone else rarely need any of the obscenely expensive blockbuster drugs these companies earn their billions from.

Thus the assumption that otherwise reasonable people may make, that your focus on keeping your carbs under control is a neurotic obsession, one step away from washing your hands 37 times a day. This is especially true in the early days after you get serious about controlling your blood sugar, when you will have to pause to look up the carb content of any food you are thinking of eating.

You may also run into trouble when people invite you to dinner and ask you what you can't eat, if you tell them that what you can't eat is a lot of sugar and *starch*. Most people nowadays are aware that people with diabetes have a "sugar problem." But it is astounding how many otherwise intelligent, highly educated people, can't get it through their heads that starch is just a string of glucose molecules. Try to explain that plates piled high with pasta, oatmeal, and healthy whole grains all turn into just as much sugar when digested as a big slice of chocolate cake and you are likely to get "that look." You may just have to learn to live with it.

Some of the people who tell you that you are making too big a deal out of your diabetes will add that they know lots of people with diabetes who are doing fine just taking their pills and eating whatever they want. I know lots of them too. I've dined with diabetic friends who take their daily pills and shot of basal insulin, then happily polish off plates piled high with pasta topped with a sugary low fat sauce. For dessert they might have a slice of sugar-free cake topped with fat-free cool whip. They aren't dead yet, and probably won't be for quite a while. Diabetes take decades to do its dirty work, just like smoking.

But "doing fine" isn't something an outsider can easily measure. High blood sugar can erode your energy levels and pack on pound after pound until it affects your mobility. Those people who look just fine might have failing kidneys and iffy hearts. Since their doctors expect this to happen to everyone with Type 2 diabetes and don't have a cure for either condition, they may just prescribe some pills and not say a whole lot about why.

The saddest thing is when I meet people in daily life who are struggling with their Type 2 Diabetes but take one look at me and assume that I can't possibly know anything that might help them because they, too, think I don't "look like someone with diabetes."

Someday I hope that the look of diabetes will be the look of the group of us people with diabetes from the alt.support.diabetes 5% Club when we got together some years ago for a face-to-face meeting at a local cafe. None of us was obese. In fact, the heaviest person at our table was someone who didn't have diabetes. We didn't look any different from any of the other people in the cafe. That's what people with well controlled diabetes look like. That is what all people with diabetes could look like.

Why Do Friends Make Fun of My Diet?

One of the more interesting findings about obesity is that people tend to end up weighing what their friends do. But if you have been heavy for a while, and most of your friends are, too, it can feel very threatening to those friends when you get serious about changing your diet. Even though your reasons for dieting may have nothing to do with your weight, weight and diet are inextricably bound in most people's minds.

So when you start avoiding the donuts in the break room or passing on the desserts at a friend's dinner party, it can make some friends feel confronted. If your friends were attracted to your circle because they felt their weight would be accepted there since everyone was heavy, your sudden onset of dieting might feel like an outright betrayal.

Teasing may be a way of expressing the uncomfortable feeling friends get when they think you are no longer "one of us." So can attempts to make you blow the diet. If your friends also have diabetes and are in denial about it, as so often happens, or if they are anxious about their diet but determined to trust their doctors, similar conflicts can arise.

When they do, there isn't a whole lot you can do about it except to remind yourself that if your friends are real friends, they should rejoice when your efforts are successful. Still, it may be wise to examine whether something you are doing is contributing to their hostile response. Are you putting out the message that everyone else should be doing what you are doing? It's easy to feel that way when your efforts are succeeding. Are you talking about nothing except your diabetes diet? If so, try to lay back a bit. Your enthusiasm, unfortunately, can come across as being judgmental and hurtful to people who haven't reached the place where they are ready to deal with their own health issues.

Will Menopause Make My Blood Sugar Get Worse?

At menopause, as their hormone levels drop, many women become more insulin resistant. But only those who already have marginal insulin production will go on to become diabetic. Just as is the case with gestational diabetes, the stress of that additional insulin resistance just unmasks the underlying deficiency.

If you have been diagnosed with Type 2 Diabetes before menopause, you may find it a bit harder to control your blood sugars after it and you will certainly find it harder to lose weight. The latter isn't because of your diabetes. Lots of women with totally normal blood sugar also get fat after they become menopausal.

What you do need to do is to be very careful with progesterone supplementation if you decide to try hormone replacement. If you have a history of getting the irresistible munchies the week before your period when you were cycling, you may find that progesterone pills have the same effect on you—except that you will be taking them every day. If you encounter this problem, ask your gynecologist to let you take your progesterone in a different form and see if that helps.

If you have been taking conjugated estrogens in the past, a switch to estradiol, which is considered to be bioidentical and is far more effective, might also result in a slight rise in your blood sugars. The benefits might still make this worth it. Work with your meter and tweak your estrogen dose until you find one high enough to be effective but low enough not to make a serious dent in your blood sugar control. I have found that an estrogen dose far lower than what is usually prescribed does everything I need.

How Can I Keep a Hospital Stay From Becoming a Nightmare?

My one overnight hospital stay since my diagnosis was a total nightmare. But it was very helpful for my readers, because that experience taught me just how dangerous a hospital can be for people with diabetes.

I had gone to the hospital because I'd inhaled a small piece of peanut, not because I had any symptom of a heart attack. Unfortunately I made the mistake of saying my chest hurt, which it did after 24 straight hours of coughing. So the first lesson I learned was this: Never say your chest hurts in an Emergency Room unless you think you could be having a heart attack. That unfortunate answer turned into $1,100 worth of medical bills.

My stay taught me that hospitals continue to force people with a diabetes diagnosis to eat the outdated high carb/ low fat diabetes diets that make it impossible to maintain anything approaching normal blood sugars. My local hospital bragged it offered a "carb reduced" diabetic menu, but what I was given for breakfast was dry toast with sugar-free jelly and fat-free scrambled eggs made out of dried powder. These people just don't get it and probably never will.

I was using mealtime insulin at the time, but was not allowed to keep my own pen. Instead a nurse measured my blood sugar with a meter that was off by some 25 mg/dl compared to my own meter. Having done that, she brought out a syringe with the thickest needle I'd ever seen with which she prepared to give me the dose of insulin she had decided I should have. I fended her off and was able to escape shortly afterward by checking myself out against medical advice. But this isn't an option if you have something serious that needs to be treated.

Appealing to the doctor who had been assigned to my care didn't help, either. As a cost saving "improvement" nowadays your own doctor doesn't come to see you in the hospital like they used to. Instead you are at the mercy of some stranger, the "hospitalist" doctor, who doesn't know a thing about you and may not even have access to your medical records. The one I was assigned to was a big fan of low fat diets for people with diabetes. She also believed that because I had a diabetes diagnosis in my medical record, I must have heart disease. Even though the expensive tests they ordered showed I did not, she worked very hard to talk me into an extremely expensive, highly invasive procedure that, had I not refused it, would probably have ended up with me getting a stent.

So if you have diabetes and there is any chance you will be in the hospital for more than a day or two, you need to be prepared with a letter signed by your doctor which states that you have maintained excellent blood sugar control for X number of years and should be allowed to choose your meals from a normal menu, not the hospital's diabetic menu. If you use insulin, your doctor should state that as long as you are conscious and rational you should be allowed to keep your own paraphernalia and to administer your own insulin.

If you are not capable of making your own decisions, you will be stuck with whatever they do to you. About the only upside to all this is that cost cutting by insurance companies has forced hospitals to send people home with indecent haste. Even procedures like gall bladder surgery are now considered day surgery, and unless something goes badly wrong, you will be sent home in time for dinner.

The only good thing about having a diabetes diagnosis when facing surgery in a hospital, I learned, is that they will schedule you for the first slot of the day because you won't be able to eat before the surgery. That's because people with poorly controlled diabetes will usually see their blood sugars rise very high when they fast. With that early slot, you are more likely to be able to go home without an overnight stay. If you aren't well enough to leave, a day or two of hospital food and Nurse Ratched's big needles won't kill you. If you can eat, get a friend or family member to bring you something appetizing and healthy when they visit.

How Do I Deal with Diabetes in a Nursing Home?

If you are forced to move to a nursing home, you won't have any control over your diet or your diabetes. A doctor's letter might help, but it might also be ignored as you get switched to the care of the doctor who supervises treatment at the nursing home. Hint: these are not always the most skillful, in-demand doctors in your community.

If you are permanently housed in a nursing home because you are in the last stages of life with dementia, there is no real point in fighting for anything but the right of your loved ones to bring you delicious foods to eat. Tight control will not make much difference at that stage of life.

But if your brain still works and your problems are only with your body, be sure you have educated your family about what diabetes-related issues are worth fighting for. Written instructions are the best, especially when signed by your doctor. So write up what you want to be fed, what medications you will and will not take, and make sure whoever will make health care decisions should you be unable to make them for yourself has a copy of this letter.

Can I Avoid A Continuous Care Community's Diabetes Diet?

The key thing to remember about assisted living facilities and nursing homes is that their Prime Directive is "Thou Shalt Not Get Sued." No institution was ever sued for feeding inmates with diabetes a low fat/high carbohydrate ADA approved diabetes diet, and therein lies the rub.

That's why I'd suggest that before you commit to moving to any facility that offers any kind of quasi-medical services, you get it in writing from the person trying to convince you to buy in that you will not be forced to eat what their nutritionist defines as a "diabetes diet" no matter what diagnoses appear on your health records.

Make sure you get a letter from your doctor like the one just mentioned in the previous section that also states that you have excellent control as a result of the diet choices you have made for decades and that you should be given total freedom to determine what you want to eat.

If you use insulin at meals, it would be nice if you could get a guarantee in writing that you will be allowed to determine your own insulin doses at mealtime, unless a doctor certifies that you are not competent to do this anymore. But there is a high probability the facility won't agree to this. Most if not all assisted living facilities and all nursing homes require that a nurse dole out any medications. This is completely understandable. They could be sued if you forget you have taken your medication and take it again.

So if you are moving somewhere that insists that a nurse give you your insulin, get it in writing that your insulin must be dosed using the specific insulin/carbohydrate ratio(s) you have found work best for you. A doctor's letter is essential here. Ask if it is possible for the nurse to let you inject yourself while she watches. And if that isn't possible, ask that the nurse give you your shot with your own ultra thin needles. Many health facilities use huge, thick, very painful needles to administer insulin to protect the staff from the possibility of getting needle sticks that could give them AIDS or hepatitis.

If the facility won't bend on these requirements, you now know what you are going to be up against. Think long and hard before moving to such a place voluntarily, even if you are moving to the independent living section. You might not be living so independently in a few years, and if you are forced to eat a diet that worsens your control and are deprived of the tools that let you maintain it, you may find yourself far more exhausted and ill than you need to be.

My Loved One Won't Take Care of Their Diabetes

Watching someone you care about ignore their diabetes is like watching them drink themselves to death or shoot heroin. And unfortunately, your ability to help them is as limited as that of the loved ones of people with fatal alcohol or drug addictions.

This isn't because uncontrolled diabetes is an addictive state. It isn't. People who have been out of control for years who finally figure out they need to cut way back on their carbs usually feel much better, not worse, which is what a recovering addict would feel.

But what the conditions have in common is that the only person who can change the self-destructive behavior involved is the person themselves. All you can do is give them the facts and then stand back. If you make controlling their blood sugars something they are supposed to do for you, watch out. A power struggle is about to develop, one that you are almost certain to lose.

So what I usually suggest to people who are facing this issue with someone they love is this: Give them the "How to Lower Your Blood Sugar Flyer," from **http://www.bloodsugar101.com/how.php**. Buy them an inexpensive meter and 100 strips at Walmart if they don't already have one. Suggest they try the technique described in the flyer for a few days. Then get out of the way.

Many people will have a moment of total revelation when they see how big a difference they have made in their blood sugar simply by cutting 50 or 60 grams of carbs out of each meal. This is so empowering, it might be all they need to break them out of the depression and despair that has kept them from taking action until now.

If you think that shame about their inability to control their weight or appetite is what is making your loved one ignore their diabetes point them to the page on the Blood Sugar 101 website that explains "You Did NOT Eat Your Way to Diabetes: The REAL Causes," found at **http://www.phlaunt.com/diabetes/14046739.php**. I have heard from quite a few people who wrote me that they were sitting with tears streaming down their face after reading that page, because until that moment they really did believe that they had given themselves an inevitably fatal condition through their own disgusting gluttony and sloth.

Self-hatred is what lies behind a lot of denial. The knowledge that it was abnormal blood sugars that led to the hunger they found so hard to control often gives people the energy they need to do what they have to do to get back into good control.

If your loved one finds the advice and information you shared with them useful and asks you further questions, keep your replies brief. Point them to online resources. Again, you want to make sure that getting control of diabetes does not turn into your thing, not theirs. It has to become their thing because they are the one who has to do all the work.

Very few people with diabetes eat perfectly, and your loved one with diabetes isn't likely to be an exception. So you don't want them to feel afraid to eat anything off-plan in front of you. If they are afraid you will judge them, it may have the paradoxical effect of making them more likely to sneak off and gorge on high carb junk where you can't see them.

I eat my share of high carb junk and I always have, throughout all the 19 years I've been dealing with diabetes. I just make sure that the amount of time I spend eating sensibly is far more than the time I spend enjoying the stuff that pushes my blood sugar up above my targets.

Remember, too, that the world today is full of health cranks who will talk your loved ones ear off about miracle supplements, exotic ingredients, and unsustainable extreme diets they are sure will cure their diabetes. These cranks do this even though none of them has diabetes or has even ever measured their own blood sugars. Because your loved one with diabetes hears too much of this kind of "helpful advice," you have to be careful not to get lumped in with all those know-it-alls. So go easy.

It can be frustrating. But you can only do what you can do. If you can't do as much as you wish you could, take a deep breath and turn your attention towards helping those who already know they need help. That is why I put my energy into building my website and writing my books. The people who come to the site are people who already know they need to do something about their diabetes and are looking for help. Over the years enough of them have contacted me to tell me how my advice has helped them that I feel grateful to have found a way to make a difference.

But people I meet face-to-face rarely want help or are willing to take advice from a friend, including me—especially since I don't "look like I have diabetes." Most of them trust their doctors or haven't reached the point where they feel the need to take charge of their health. So when I'm with them, we talk about other things. If they ever do decide they want to check out what I'm into, they know where my website is. But each of us can only do so much for other people. Even those we deeply love.

Chapter Seven

How Can I Get My Doctor to Be More Helpful?

Why Is My Doctor That Way?

To understand why it can be so difficult to get your family doctor to give you the help you need when you are working to achieve normal, healthy blood sugar levels, you have to relate to the conditions under which that doctor has to practice.

Family doctors, a.k.a. primary care providers (PCPs), treat several thousand patients each year. To do their jobs right, they have to know a little bit about every medical condition a patient might walk in with. That way they can recognize emergencies, determine whether a patient should be sent to a specialist, and know enough to be able to order the proper tests that lead to a correct diagnosis.

Since there are hundreds of medical conditions they must keep track of ranging from abdominal aortic aneurism to zygomycosis, family doctors concentrate, quite rightly, on recognizing and diagnosing the conditions that could quickly become an emergency.

If your symptoms or test results suggest you might have something serious you will usually get immediate attention. Your family doctor will refer you to a specialist right away and may even call the specialist's office themselves to ensure you get a timely appointment.

Family doctors are very good at this. I've had one call up an ophthalmologist on a Sunday morning, who met me at his office an hour later just so he could make sure my retinas were still where they were supposed to be, despite the flashing lights I was seeing. (They were, thank goodness.) Years ago, another family doctor phoned the ER at our local hospital so they could have a team waiting to treat my toddler when he had a dramatic symptom that might have been caused by a very dangerous bacterial infection that could have permanently crippled him. (It wasn't. He had a virus that caused the identical symptom.)

But family doctors don't consider Type 2 Diabetes an emergency. Not when they are dealing every day with patients who have virulent infections, fast growing cancers, ectopic pregnancies, and carotid arteries that are 97% blocked by plaque. Yes, diabetes causes all kinds of nasty and crippling outcomes, but not for another decade or two.

Beside that, as you read earlier, doctors have been trained to believe that you could prevent your diabetes if you'd only lose weight and that, if you won't, there really isn't a whole lot they can do to keep those bad outcomes from occurring in that distant future. So when you show up for your appointment, your diabetes is very low on the list of things your doctor has to worry about. They will treat it just as they do all the other chronic conditions their patients may have that they manage.

The way your doctor manages all the hundreds of chronic conditions their patients may have is by following the official practice guidelines for each of these chronic conditions. These guidelines are formal documents published by committees of doctors who are specialists in each condition. Since primary care doctors don't have the time to follow the research about all the chronic conditions they manage, they rely on the practice guidelines these experts publish to tell them exactly what tests they should order, what test results require further action, and what drugs a family doctor should prescribe before a patient needs to see a specialist for more advanced treatment. There are separate practice guidelines published for dozens of chronic conditions, be they COPD, ulcers, arthritis, psoriasis, kidney disease, heart disease, or depression.

Unfortunately for us, the organization that writes the practice guidelines for treating Type 2 Diabetes in the United States is our old friend, the American Diabetes Association — the ADA. There are other organizations around the world who also publish guidelines, most notably, the World Health Organization (WHO), but most of these other organizations just copy the guidelines the ADA comes out with.

I say unfortunately, because the ADA's treatment recommendations are based on its long-defended belief that people with Type 2 Diabetes are fine with A1Cs below 8.0%. Their guidelines state that the appropriate treatment for Type 2 Diabetes is to start patients off with metformin and then, if their A1Cs are still above 8.0%, add one after the other of the latest, expensive patented drugs to the patient's daily regimen until an A1C in the 7% range has been achieved.

Only after all the oral drugs and the expensive patented injected non-insulin drugs have failed to lower the A1C below 8%, does the ADA recommend that insulin be prescribed. Even then they only suggest that doctors prescribe basal insulin, the kind that only lowers fasting blood sugar but doesn't do much to prevent very high post-meal blood sugars spikes. This remains true, even though there is quite a bit of research that suggests that the best drug for someone recently diagnosed with diabetes is fast-acting insulin, the kind used to lower blood sugars at mealtimes, even when used for only a few weeks or months.

It gets worse. The ADA also continues to tell doctors that achieving a post-meal blood sugar below 180 mg/dl {10} is what they call "tight control" and goes on to explain that tight control is too difficult for most patients to attain. So the message most family doctors get is that post-meal blood sugars can be ignored.

And then, to top it off, as mentioned earlier, the ADA continues to insist that people with diabetes can eat all the foods other people can, but should try to eat a "healthy" diet—that low fat, high carb diet full of bananas, oatmeal, and lots of whole grain bread.

Those of us who have watched the ADA resolutely refuse to inform doctors that diets that significantly lower carbohydrates are more effective than any drug currently on the market, assume this refusal has something to do with who provides the bulk of the money that keeps the ADA funded: the big drug companies and the mass market packaged food companies.

But like it or not, these practice guidelines are all your busy doctor may know about diabetes. So when you walk into the office upset about your post-meal blood sugar spikes up to 260 mg//dl {14.4}, your doctor pulls out your most recent blood test sees that your A1C is 6.8% and that there's no protein in your urine. They then take your blood pressure, which is fine, check out your retinas which are clear, and decide that you are not only not an emergency waiting to happen, but that you don't need any treatment at all, since the ADA's guidelines describe you as already being in "very good control." This means there's no reason for them to waste any more of their precious time on you.

And their time is precious, given how many patients they have to see each day. Precious, and constantly being wasted by people they politely refer to as "the worried well"—and privately by something less printable. These are the people who have been to three specialists already but still insist that the pain from their ingrown toenail is cancer or that an attack of sneezing means they have AIDS. They annoy doctors because they take up valuable time that could have been used to treat people with real problems. Doctors would rather spend their precious time getting approval from an insurance company for the rare and expensive drug that could keep a young mother alive instead

156 ❖ Your Diabetes Questions Answered

of debating, with a member of the worried well, the dangers of eating wheat.

So when you launch into the speech where you ask your doctor to help you bring your 6.8% A1C down into the 5% range and try to explain why you are so upset by those highs after meals, here's what happens: Your doctor, who has never read anything about the impact of high post-meal blood sugars on health, since they aren't mentioned in the practice guidelines, starts thinking, "Great blood sugar control. No complications. Another time wasting hypochondriac," and their bedside manner shifts into the "get her out of the office" protocol.

It gets worse if you make the mistake of pulling out a research study you found on the web. The worried well include many people who visit alternative medicine websites and come into the office brandishing research studies they downloaded from these sites, most of them published in the vanity journals we discussed on Page 108. This is the "tin foil hat contingent." They are even more persistent than the average hypochondriac and your doctor hates them. They don't want to read the thoroughly debunked studies these people insist prove that vaccines cause autism or that fluoridation causes cancer, dementia, or mental deficiency in children. They don't have the time to explain why the *Journal of Nutraceuticals* is not a legitimate source of medical information and they know from long experience that no matter what they might say, the tin foil hat contingent won't believe a word of it.

So the minute you start to mention your totally relevant study published in high quality journals like *Diabetes Care* or even the *New England Journal of Medicine* your doctor will invoke the "tin foil hat protocol." Then, before you know it, you are standing at the checkout desk, being booked for a follow-up visit six months hence—and seething.

I used to think very bad thoughts about doctors who dismissed my concerns and refused to listen to what I had learned in my research. But after establishing my Blood Sugar 101 website I have received so much mail from the worried well and the tinfoil hat contingent that I've begun to understand why doctors are the way they are.

These people write 1,000 word emails about how worried they are that their blood sugars spike to 108 after eating and how sure they are that this is why their arm is always hurting. Assuring them they are normal provokes a 2,000 word rebuttal. Others send study after vanity journal study—all full-text—promoting obscure supplements that come attached to emails demanding that I read and comment on them.

The truly needy people I hear from usually begin by apologizing for taking up my time. The worried well and the tin foil hat contingent get offended when I don't read and comment on the three months worth of blood sugar logs they sent me.

So that is what your doctor is up against. If you realize it and are gentle with them, over time, you may be able to find a way to get them to give you the help you need.

Are Endocrinologists More Helpful?

Unlike your family doctor, your endocrinologist specializes in the treatment of diabetes, so you could be forgiven for thinking that they keep up with the latest research by reading journal articles and thinking through their implications. But you'd be wrong.

Your endocrinologist spent many very expensive years training in endocrinology and during that period they probably did read everything they could. But those years are far in the past. Since beginning their practice the endo has been seeing patients around the clock and is far too burnt out to do anything more than read the newsletters, funded by drug companies, that summarize the high points of what the latest new drugs do. Occasionally they highlight side effects recently discovered in older drugs that are now off patent and available in cheap generic versions that compete with the expensive new drugs.

Every now and then endos go to conferences where they hear presentations given by famous endocrinologists, almost all of whom are on drug company payrolls. Like every other doctor ever surveyed, these rock star endos are convinced that they remain completely objective despite the tens of thousands of dollars they receive every year from drug companies in the form of speaking fees and travel expenses to glamorous destinations. They adhere to this belief, though study after study has documented that doctors who take so much as a ball point pen or a free lunch from a drug company rep become more likely to prescribe the drugs the rep promotes.

Though endocrinologists are specialists, unless you are very lucky, the endo you visit is likely to follow the exact same practice recommendations in treating your Type 2 Diabetes as your family doctor follows until your A1C is north of 9.0% or 10%. At that point an endo may prescribe some special formulations of basal insulin that are helpful to people with extreme insulin resistance or a fast-acting insulin to be used at mealtime. These are too complicated for family doctors to deal with.

Remember, too, that when you wander into an endocrinologist's office, most of the diabetic patients they see regularly have Type 1 Diabetes, which is extremely challenging to manage. When they do see people with Type 2 diabetes, they have usually been referred because they have A1Cs north of 10%. You aren't likely to get the help you hope for if you come in hoping to lower your A1C from 6.8% to a completely normal level.

The endo may be even less patient with you than your family doctor was. In their mind, you are wasting time that could have been spent helping a teenager fresh from the ER where they were just diagnosed with Type 1 Diabetes after testing with a blood sugar of 580 mg/dl {32.2} or working out the insulin doses needed by a veteran whose uncontrolled diabetes has already lead to the amputation of three toes.

There are occasional exceptions—endocrinologists who are more open to offering you support. In my experience, they may be doctors who have just opened up new practices and need to fill up their schedules with anyone whose insurance will pay for a visit. But there are far fewer endocrinologists in the United States and elsewhere than there are patients who need them. So it's normal to have to wait three to six months to get an appointment and even more normal to come away from that appointment without having gotten much help if your A1C hasn't reached alarming heights.

Even if an endo agrees to take you on as a patient when you are in good control, after the first appointment you may be handed over to the care of a Nurse Practitioner, who will never deviate from the practice guidelines, because without an MD degree that is all they are allowed to do.

That's why I wouldn't suggest seeing an endocrinologist unless there is a good possibility your "Type 2 Diabetes" diagnosis is wrong and you have autoimmune diabetes (a form of Type 1) or something even more obscure or when your blood sugars have not come down in response to a low carb diet, metformin, and basal insulin.

What's the Best Way to Ask for a Doctor's Help?

Now that you have a better idea of how your doctors are likely to perceive you, you can better understand what the best strategies are for coping with them. The basic principles are simple:

Make it fast. Your doctor wants you out of the office to make room for people with more critical problems. So come to the appointment with a small list of what you want the doctor to do for you. Remember your doctor's services are limited to ordering tests or prescribing drugs. That's what doctors do. Don't expect your doctor to know much about the drugs they prescribe. The people who understand drugs are the registered pharmacists attached to the pharmacy where you get your drugs. They are the people to talk with about whether a drug you might want to try will interact badly with other drugs you take and to ask about serious potential side effects or other reasons you might want to avoid the drug. Doctors rarely keep up with information about the drugs they prescribe, but pharmacists do If they don't know something, they will look it up and get back to you. Limit the topics you discuss with your doctor to a few important issues.

2. **Make it simple.** If you want medical tests, be very clear about what condition you want to be tested for and, if you know the names of the tests, ask for the specific tests you'd like to have. If you want prescriptions, have them in a list by name. Check your insurance company's drug formulary or call customer service before your appointment to be sure that the tests and drugs you need are covered by your insurance without the need for prior authorization. Prior authorization requires your doctor to fill out time-consuming forms and to explain in writing why you can't use the other, cheaper medications or tests the insurer covers. Don't expect a doctor to do this for you if they think you are already in fine shape.

3. **Respect your doctor's reasons for refusing what you ask for and listen closely to those reasons.** Often there are things in your medical record that might make a drug dangerous for you. Or in the case of tests, you may already have had tests that rule out what the test you are asking for can diagnose. For example, if you have had a C-peptide test that shows you are producing insulin in the amounts typical of Type 2 Diabetes, there is no need for the fasting insulin test or an antibody test used to diagnose autoimmune diabetes. Don't get hostile or suggest your doctor is ignorant if what you ask for is denied. If you really disagree with the doctor's reasoning, you'll have to find another doctor.

4. **Show up with convincing blood sugar levels.** You won't get help with a good A1C. If you've been controlling with a stringent ketogenic diet, and are burning out on eating no more than 45 grams a day, you may hope that using insulin will make it possible to eat more carbs and still hit your blood sugar targets, which it would. But your ultra low carb, ketogenic diet will have lowered your A1C 2, 3, or even 4% from where it would be had you been eating all that whole wheat bread, bananas, and oatmeal most people with Type 2 Diabetes are told to eat. So if you go into your appointment with an A1C below 7.5% even though it would have been an A1C of 10% without that ketogenic diet, you will get no help at all.

That's because most doctors and even many endocrinologists have no idea what a dramatic effect cutting carbs has on blood sugar levels. So it's a waste of time to explain that your 6.2% A1C was achieved by eating less than 15 grams of carbohydrate per meal. Your doctor won't understand that without eating at that extremely low carbohydrate

intake level, your A1C would be at the 8.8% level where you were diagnosed. Almost every doctor who sees that 6.8% will think you are in
great control and refuse you insulin.

Reports from a lot of correspondents who have had this experience
have convinced me that with the reliance that doctors now put on the
A1C test, all you can do to get the help you need is to give up your
healthy diet for a month to six weeks and eat a ton of carbs so you can
produce an A1C high enough to get your doctor's attention. When you
do this, make sure to log your post-meal blood sugars and make sure
they are all at least in the middle 200s {i.e. 14.4} or higher. This seems
to be the only way to be taken seriously. If your meter lets you print
out a graph of your month's worth of blood sugar readings, print it
and bring it along. It's a shame people have to do this. But the tripling
of insulin prices over the past decade has made insurers much less
willing to pay for insulin, while the recent approval and heavy marketing of whole families of new, expensive, and potentially dangerous
oral drugs has made doctors less willing to prescribe insulin to anyone
with Type 2. Even so, if you need insulin to make it possible to maintain good control without eating like a monk, it is worth doing. A
month of ugly control won't ruin your health, and once you get the
prescriptions you need you can go back to eating to your meter.

5. **When you need a real expert, go where the real experts are.**
When you have a serious medical problem you can't resolve with your
local doctors, seek out younger doctors who practice out of the hospital that is associated with the best medical school in your region. These
are the doctors who graduated in the top of their class. Since they are
young, their training is more recent and they are more likely to be up-
to-date on relevant research. Example of issues that require a trip to a
distant teaching hospital endocrinologist might be:

❖ Very high blood sugars (well over 200 mg/dl {11.1}) that stay high
for much of the day and don't come down in response to a low
carb diet, pills, or the insulin you have already been prescribed.

❖ Blood sugars that are worsening from month to month even
though you haven't changed your medications or diet.

❖ Blood sugars that are completely unpredictable making it
impossible to dose mealtime insulin without experiencing hypos
when meals without insulin eventually put you into the high 200s
{15} or above.

These are conditions these doctors are trained to treat.

Why Does My Doctor Give Me Such Awful Diet Advice?

Medical school does not educate doctors about nutrition except at the very basic level where a healthy diet is defined as one low in saturated fats and filled with fruits, vegetables and whole grains. Since the ADA guidelines for years specified that people with diabetes should eat a very low fat diet due to the now discredited belief that eating fat causes heart disease and that natural fats like butter are as dangerous as trans fat, most doctors still believe that people with diabetes should eat low fat diets full of whole wheat bread, oatmeal, and sugary fruits like bananas.

It is useless to argue, because most younger doctors have completely normal blood sugars themselves and can't see the impact of carbs on their blood sugar even if they test. I get a small but significant stream of mail from older physicians recently diagnosed with Type 2 Diabetes lamenting that they had no idea how flawed the advice was that they had been giving their patients until they had to test their own diabetic blood sugar and saw the impact of those supposedly healthy low fat/high carb fruits and grains.

Doctors won't take for advice from patients, so don't attempt to instruct them. I have yet to have a doctor ask me how I have managed to keep my A1C in the 5% range for most of the 19 years since I've been diagnosed. I know for a fact—having seen a page of my medical records by accident—that one of my doctors thought I was imagining my diabetes, though I was able to produce a reading in the 200s on command. (All it took was eating a single small "healthy whole grain and fruit muffin" and heading to the lab an hour later.)

Your doctor is useful for ordering the tests you need to monitor your progress and prescribing the drugs you may need to maintain it. Beyond that, you are mostly on your own.

This is why I have dedicated so much of my time over the last decade to posting what I've learned on the my website where people who need this kind of information can find it. I'm very glad that they do. Even quite a few doctors and nurses have found it helpful—but only after their own diagnoses have taught them how bad the advice in the ADA guidelines really is.

My Doctor Won't Prescribe the Drugs I Need What Should I Do?

It's important to listen to the reasons why your doctor won't prescribe. To be honest, this is often the sign of a competent doctor, because, in my experience, the least competent ones are the ones most likely to be influenced by drug salespeople and prescribe every new drug as soon as it hits the market, even though at that point most of its side effects are as yet completely unknown.

The better doctors I've seen always prefer to prescribe older, well-understood drugs in non-critical situations. If you were battling an otherwise fatal cancer, they might suggest you sign up to try something highly experimental with possibly devastating side effects, but a good doctor won't give you a brand new drug for diabetes unless you are running the A1Cs above 10.0% they consider an emergency and have already tried everything else.

Doctors will also be very resistant to prescribing meal-time insulin nowadays because using it safely requires that someone give you some training, which they don't have the resources to provide. People with Type 1 get this expensive training because insurers will pay for it. But that's because they can die without insulin. You won't.

By the same token, it's almost impossible for someone with Type 2 to get an insulin pump or a continuous glucose monitor covered by insurance even though these could be very helpful. These devices are just too expensive. Insurers can't afford to cover them for the millions of people with Type 2 Diabetes. The only way you can get them is to have very good insurance and a doctor who is willing to battle through the reams of paperwork it takes. Usually you need to have a history of multiple hospitalizations for severe hypos before a doctor will be willing to start the process.

If you plan to pay for your own devices and their very expensive consumables, make sure your doctor knows this, as it may make them more comfortable prescribing. But check out the prices first. Most devices are many thousands of dollars a year. Insulin not covered by your insurance can be exorbitant, too, and many insurers are limiting which brands of insulins they will cover. So before you ask for insulin, research which brands your plan will cover. If you don't, your doctor may be faced with the need to write letters to insurers they just don't have the time to write.

Why Did My Doctor Warn Me an A1C Below 6.5% Is Dangerous?

Unfortunately, a large study of people with Type 2 Diabetes who strove to get their A1Cs under 6.5% was published in 2008 that came to the conclusion that people who lowered their A1Cs to that level were more likely to have heart attacks than those who didn't. This was the ACCORD study. It attracted a huge amount of attention in the medical press.

This was a classic case of poorly interpreted results. Further analyses of the data from which the original conclusion was drawn found that the people who actually had had the excess heart attacks were *not* the people who had lowered their A1Cs below 6.5%. They were the people assigned to the group who were supposed to try to reach that goal but did not reach it. It also turned out that people who had the excess heart attacks had been taking Avandia, a drug now known to raise the risk of heart attacks.

Another large, much less well publicized study, ADVANCE, which also examined what happened when people brought their A1Cs down below 6.5% was published a year or so earlier and got almost no press. It did not detect any excess heart attacks in people who lowered their A1Cs, just significant health benefits. Not so coincidentally, none of the people in this study were taking Avandia.

But most doctors only read about the ACCORD results that were in the headlines of all the newsletters doctors follow. They never saw the subgroup analyses that explained who really got those heart attacks. So many doctors now believe that it is proven science that lowering your A1C to a level that is still considerably higher than normal — 6.4% — is, for mysterious reasons, very dangerous for people with Type 2 Diabetes. Some will take away your prescriptions if your A1C drops to that level. Some will lecture you severely about the dangers of lowering your A1C, even if you do it with diet alone, even though all the participants in the ACCORD study were all taking a cocktail of three or four drugs, which they needed because they were eating those low fat/high carbohydrates diets that raise blood sugar.

There has never been a published study that looks at what happens when a large group of people with Type 2 Diabetes attempt to lower their A1Cs using carb restriction and only a few safe drugs.

If you do have the misfortune to see a doctor who is still giving out this toxic and mistaken advice or who berates you for letting your A1C drop below 6.5%, there is no point in trying to change their mind. Doctors will never listen to people who aren't doctors when it comes to medical information. Find a different doctor who will support you attaining your goals. They do exist.

Why Did My Doctor Tell Me That People over 65 Don't Need to Keep Their A1Cs Under 8%?

This is a recent, very disturbing, addition to the guidelines doctors and insurers follow. The reasoning behind it is that as we explained earlier, hypos are more dangerous for older people than they are for the young. Frequent hypos can damage older people's brains and shorten their lives.

So the authorities who write guidelines have decided that it is safer to keep old people's blood sugars up in the range where hypos aren't as likely to occur rather than risk them having those hypos. Keeping your blood sugars above 183 mg/dl most of the time, which is what it takes to get an 8.0% A1C will do that. After all—the subtext seems to go—these people have a disease we know will shorten their lifespan, so they probably won't live long enough to develop the complications these higher blood sugars will cause.

And of course, the insurers and government health plans love this guideline because it saves them a ton of money on drugs and insulin.

Obviously, this guideline makes sense if the older person in question is frail, suffering from diminished reasoning powers and/or memory, or living with other health conditions that are likely to shorten their lives. But it is tragically misguided when applied to healthy, active people over 65 who are eating a diet that keeps their blood sugars in a normal or near normal range, who could easily live to be a hundred.

Sadly, many older people with diabetes, who have blindly followed their doctors' orders for years and never made the effort to really understand their condition, think it is good news when they are told, in effect, to stop worrying about their blood sugar. They may see this as permission to eat what they want, stop taking insulin, and give up buying the much-too-expensive oral drugs they have been taking to control their blood sugars.

But if you don't feel that way, you have every right to demand that your doctors respect that you are competent and capable enough to continue using the drugs and diet that work for you and that they support your efforts to keep your blood sugars under tight control. If you do not have a history of having hypos, there is no reason to be any less aggressive with your diabetes regimen.

How Can I Tell If I Have a Competent Doctor?

It is only when we get a diagnosis of a serious illness that most of us learn whether our doctors really are competent. Until then, we tend to rate our doctors by how friendly they are and whether they seem to care about us. But the world is full of very friendly doctors whose healthy patients adore them and recommend them to friends who are dangerous if you have something serious wrong with you.

That sounds harsh, but after a very nice, helpful, friendly doctor told me to ignore what turned out to be an early melanoma, I heartily believe it. Another very personable doctor I used to see missed appendicitis in a friend's child resulting in a burst appendix. I have heard from hundreds of people over the years whose friendly, helpful doctors have given them appallingly bad treatment for their diabetes, treatment that led them to develop the kind of very serious complications that nobody who is getting regular medical care should ever experience today.

Far better to find a grumpy doctor with no bedside manner who knows what they are doing—though there are plenty of grumpy doctors who are incompetent too.

At a minimum your doctor should:

❖ Support you in your desire to attain normal or near normal blood sugars, not just the "good enough for a person with diabetes" blood sugars that lead to complications.

❖ Never tell you that it is dangerous to achieve A1Cs in the 5% range unless you are doing it by using insulin or insulin stimulating drugs in ways that are causing you to experience frequent hypos.

❖ Never take away the medications that give you good control when you finally attain it.

❖ Periodically run the tests all people with diabetes should have, like the microalbumin test that will let you know if you have early kidney disease and the test for vitamin B12 that anyone taking metformin should get after they have taken that drug for four years or longer.

❖ Support you when you request a prescription for a drug you feel will help you lower your blood sugar or give you an explanation you can understand about why that drug might be a bad choice for someone with your health history.

❖ Support you when you refuse to take a drug that you have good reason to believe might not be as safe as the drug companies say it is. The best doctors are much more cautious about prescribing any new drug than the incompetent ones.

❖ Trust you when you report that your blood sugars have become impossible to control and not accuse you overtly or by implication of lying about taking your medications or sticking to your diet.

❖ Give you a referral to a highly trained endocrinologist at a teaching hospital if you are having serious difficulty controlling your blood sugar with the insulin they prescribe, rather than insisting you see the guy they golf with, who practices out of the local, fourth rate community hospital

❖ Trust you when you report that you are seeing much higher blood sugars on your meter than your A1C test results predict and be aware that there are genetic variants that make the A1C test yield dangerously misleading results.

Note: A small number of doctors in the U.S. — mostly in California — are paid a flat amount each year to care for each patient using a reimbursement plan called "capitation." Some plans are structured so that the doctor earns more if their patients use fewer medical services than expected. If you are having trouble getting tests or other services you need, ask your doctor if they are being paid a flat rate to provide your care. If the answer is "yes," ask to have the plan explained. If the doctor can't or won't explain it, it might be time to find another doctor.

Will Weight Loss Surgery Cure My Diabetes?

Weight loss surgery has been very heavily promoted as a miracle cure for diabetes by the surgeons who profit mightily from performing it. Since there is no agency that regulates surgery the way that the FDA regulates drugs, surgeons can get away with making the most extreme claims without having to prove they are true.

What research we do have about the effect of weight loss surgery on diabetes suggests that like every other "cure" for diabetes, it mainly works by forcing people to stop eating the carbs that raise their blood sugars. People whose diabetes is caused by an inability to secrete insulin will not see their diabetes cured by weight loss surgery. And people who have the surgery, whose blood sugars improve, often see them rise back into the diabetic range as soon as their surgically-altered stomachs stretch back out to where they can eat a lot more.

So be very cautious before you let anyone persuade you that weight loss surgery is anything more than a very expensive, though effective, way to force you to stop eating more than a few teaspoons of food per meal. It isn't a cure for anything but overeating. If you can find a less dangerous way to cut back on how much carbohydrate you eat, you may be able to achieve the same degree of "diabetes reversal" without undergoing surgery. Weight loss surgery profoundly alters how your digestive system works, permanently. It also has a small but significant chance of killing you.

Chapter Eight
Should I Take This Drug?

Isn't It Better to Control Without Any Drugs?

It would be wonderful if you could get perfect blood sugars by making a few simple changes to your diet and then sticking to that diet for the next fifty years. There are people who do this and my hat is off to them. But lots of us can't, including a lot of people who are very careful about what they eat.

The years of exposure to high blood sugars that occur before you get a diagnosis may have taken a hard toll on your beta cells. It's commonly stated that people with Type 2 Diabetes will have lost between 50% and 80% of their beta cells by the time of their diagnosis. They rarely grow back, even when we prevent further damage from occurring.

So even a very strict low carb diet may not be enough to give you the near normal blood sugars you need to preserve your health. Even if it does, it may require you to eat a diet so stringent it's impossible to stick to it for more than a few years, because you burnout on how many foods are forbidden. Other times you may find that even a ketogenic diet is still letting your blood sugars roller-coaster enough to make you still get hungry. Very low carb diets can also make your energy levels may tank due to subtle changes in how the thyroid works that sometimes occur in people who have been eating ketogenic diets for a long time.

When diet doesn't work as hoped, you may feel like a failure. The people who do well on these diets are so vocal online, that when you don't do well on one, you may think it's your fault. You may also assume that the people who can stick to these diets have more moral fiber than you do.

But my long years of interacting with people with Type 2 Diabetes have convinced me that the people who stay well controlled with diet alone aren't virtuous. They are just people whose metabolisms are such that it is much easier for them to eat a diet that completely controls their blood sugar. Their energy levels are as good or better on a very low carb diet than they are when eating more carbs, and they are often large enough, young enough, or male enough, to be able to maintain excellent blood sugar control eating a lot more grams of carbohydrate per meal—and a lot more food, period--than those of us who struggle. Some just don't care that much about what they eat and don't feel deprived eating the same foods day after day as they don't get all that much pleasure out of eating.

So if you find that your diet is no longer working, for whatever reason, don't waste time beating yourself up for not being perfect. Call for the reinforcements, in the form of safe drugs.

I learned this the hard way. For years I was determined to manage my diabetes without drugs because I had already suffered a serious, permanent side effect after taking a prescription drug. But I have an insulin sensitive form of diabetes where my blood sugars rise because my pancreas doesn't secrete insulin properly. My blood sugars would spike over 140 mg/dl {7.8} if I ate more than 15 grams of carbohydrate at once, and over time my energy levels dropped to where I felt like dead meat most of the time.

After five years of obsessional strictness, punctuated in the middle by a year of total burnout, I decided to try the metformin my doctor offered. Metformin helped control my hunger but did little for my blood sugars, because my problem wasn't insulin resistance, just poor insulin secretion. After metformin failed, my doctor suggested I try Avandia. (This was before the news about its heart attack side effect was made public) It didn't do a thing for my blood sugar either. It was only after I found an endo willing to let me try fast-acting insulin at meals that my blood sugars leveled out and I started feeling good again.

It was a revelation! I felt like a drooping plant that had finally been watered. My energy level rose, and much to my doctors' surprise I lost a couple of pounds without trying. That's when I realized how much unnecessary suffering I'd caused myself by being so determined to avoid all drugs. Had any diet made me feel as good as that insulin did, I would have had no problem sticking to it.

Mealtime Insulin isn't easy to use, so I was still having to keep a close eye on what I ate, but the extra 20 or 30 grams of carb it let me eat at each meal were worth it. I didn't mind any of the effort involved because it made me feel so much better.

So now I urge people who can't control their blood sugars without eating extremely restrictive diets to try one or two of the few, well-understood, safe diabetic drugs. These are older drugs that have been in use long enough for their true effectiveness to have become better understood and for any dangerous side effects they might cause to have become known. Most of these drugs have had their patents expire so they are available in cheaper generic forms.

That's a nice plus, too—as it means you can usually get them for only a couple dollars a month. But it also offers the advantage that since the drug is no longer earning some big drug company billions, researchers at institutions heavily funded by Big Pharma are finally free to publish studies that reveal any problems with the drug that the drug companies might have been keeping hidden while it was still under patent.

And it isn't conspiracy thinking that makes me say that the drug companies use their financial clout to keep these problems hidden while a drug is earning them billions. There's plenty of evidence. After Avandia was shown to cause excess heart attacks, it emerged that the company who made it, GlaxoSmithKline, had threatened a billion dollar lawsuit against the University of North Carolina to prevent one of its doctors from publishing a study that would have revealed the heart attack-Avandia connection. The study remained unpublished. Merck intimidated a Stanford University professor who raised questions about the safety of now-withdrawn, stroke-causing drug, Vioxx. Patients only learned that statins dramatically raise the risk of developing diabetes after Lipitor lost its patent. The research confirming this was published just weeks after that patent expiration.

So some caution is in order. Avoid taking any new drug until it has been on the market at least five years. That excludes all the drugs you see in those TV commercials filled with ecstatic, middle-aged models whose delight makes them look more like partakers in medical marijuana than people suffering the dozens of side effects that the announcer chants in the speeded up monotone playing in the background.

Even five years is rarely enough time for the most significant side effects to emerge with any diabetes drug. These are drugs you may be taking every day for the next couple decades, which is far longer than anyone took the drugs during the clinical trials that were the basis for their approval. Even when the FDA stipulates that a drug company is supposed to do a follow-up long-term safety study, these studies are rarely performed. They are expensive, and the FDA doesn't impose sanctions when the studies aren't done.

So unless there is some very good reason for trying a newer drug, it's best to limit yourself to the drugs that have been on the market for longer than the 14 years that patent protection lasts. It is possible that some wonderful new drug will come along whose benefits are so great that it is worth the risk of trying it. But every time I've been snookered into thinking this might be true, and have tried and/or recommended a newish drug, some worrisome issue has emerged a few years later and I have ended up wishing I'd stuck to my own advice and left the new stuff alone.

What Drugs Are Safe?

This isn't the place to go into all the technical reasons why so many drugs aren't safe for people with Type 2 Diabetes. I've posted that information on the bloodsugar101.com website. If you want to know the details, and I hope you do, you can find many pages containing summaries of the research behind these claims and view the actual research studies by visiting the Blood Sugar 101 Drugs page.

But here's the very brief summary: The drugs I consider safe when they are prescribed with full awareness of any warnings that might appear on the drug's official, FDA approved label are listed below. These drugs are:

❖ Acarbose
❖ Metformin
❖ Repaglinide
❖ Injected basal insulin
❖ Injected fast-acting insulin.

Though they may be safe for most people with Type 2 Diabetes, there are still good reasons why a doctor might not think it a good idea for you to take any one of them. Here are some of them:

❖ Acarbose won't work unless you are still producing enough insulin two hours after eating to dispose of the carbs from a meal once it has finally digested.

❖ Metformin is not safe if you have serious kidney or liver problems.

❖ Repaglinide is not safe unless your blood sugars shoot up at least into the mid 200s {around 13} when you eat the amount of carbohydrate you plan to eat while taking it.

❖ Fast-acting insulin also is not safe if you have gastroparesis which makes it impossible to know when your blood sugar will peak after a meal. It also isn't safe unless your blood sugars rise very high without it—at least to the mid 200s {around 13}.

❖ Basal insulin can be tough to use properly unless your fasting blood sugar is closer to 160 {8.9} than 120 mg/dl {6.6}.

All the rest of the drugs that doctors may prescribe have serious drawbacks. The older, cheap drugs that stimulate insulin release, which belong to the sulfonylurea drug family, seem to raise, not lower, the risk of having a heart attack. They also cause insulin to be secreted for long stretches of time, whether or not there is food coming in. This can make you very hungry, which inevitably leads to weight gain. Because the insulin they cause to be secreted can't be turned off, they must be eaten with a very high carb diet if you are to avoid having dangerous hypos that can send you to the ER.

The newer incretin drugs like Januvia and Victoza come with a different set of problems. Though they can sometimes achieve dramatic improvements in blood sugar, there are worrisome studies that point to the fact that they may be causing permanent structural changes in the pancreas of a type that over time might destroy it or lead to the development of a fatal pancreatic cancer. Some also can cause damaging attacks of inflammation that permanently damage your joints. This is a known side effect, but one many family doctors aren't aware of. I have heard from several people who have ended up with severe joint problems after taking Januvia. They did not have any such problems before starting the drug.

The most recent class of new drugs, the SGLT-2 inhibitors like Invokana and Jardiance, are so new that many of their side effects are only starting to emerge. But those that have emerged are very troubling. They lower blood sugar by changing how your kidneys work and making them pee away excess blood glucose. It is only a few years since they hit the market, but already we have learned they can damage bone, make amputations more likely, and even cause diabetic ketoacidosis, a potentially fatal condition that until the emergence of these drugs had only been diagnosed in people with Type 1 Diabetes, never in Type 2.

Should I Try Acarbose?

Acarbose is a very rarely prescribed diabetes drug that slows down the digestion of starches and some sugars and delays the blood sugar spike they cause. It does this by keeping the body from making an enzyme needed to digest complex sugars and starches. It can be useful to people in the earlier stages of Type 2 Diabetes who still produce significant amounts of insulin a few hours after they eat.

The reason that acarbose is rarely prescribed is that if you take it and eat a normal amount of carbohydrate it will make you extremely gassy, so gassy that most people who try it decide it's better to live with higher blood sugars than become a social outcast.

But acarbose can work for people who are eating diets that are quite low in carbohydrate. When I was attempting to control with diet alone, I found I could use it if I took it once a day and only used it to cover a meal that contained an extra 20-30 grams of carbs. This was enough to let me enjoy a treat or two that otherwise would spike my blood sugar too high. But using for two meals a day—no way. The gas produced was intolerable. So if you have been eating a low carbohydrate diet for a while and want a bit more space in your diet for starches, it might be worth a try.

One thing to keep in mind is that acarbose only delays the production of blood glucose from starches and sugars that require the use of enzymes to be digested. Simple sugars like glucose itself or dextrose, which is just another name for glucose, go right into your blood stream when you eat them. So acarbose doesn't block their absorption.

What Does Metformin Do?

Metformin has been in use since it was first approved in Europe in the 1950 but it's effects are still not completely understood. What is known is that it flips a switch in muscle tissue that makes muscle cells burn glucose more efficiently. This is why metformin is usually described as "lowering insulin resistance."

It is very useful for people whose high blood sugar is mostly due to insulin resistance. If you don't respond to it at all, it can mean you don't actually have classic Type 2 Diabetes but some other form of diabetes that mostly affects your insulin supply.

Metformin also seems to stop the liver from storing and dumping glucose. This happens no matter whether you are resistant to insulin or insulin sensitive. Even people with Type 1 Diabetes benefit from this effect because blocking liver dumping will lower post-meal blood sugars independent of what is happening in your muscles.

The way metformin limits the liver's ability to store glucose may explain why it often causes people to lose a couple pounds when they first start taking it. They are probably losing the same water weight associated with stored glycogen we discussed on page 91.

Besides producing these effects on blood sugar, metformin also seems to be protective against heart attack. I've heard from a few physicians that some of their cardiologist friends take metformin even though they don't have a diagnosis of diabetes. This protective effect may be partially because it lowers undiagnosed high post-meal blood sugars—the ones we know can cause changes in the arteries that lead to heart disease. But it also appears to change the way heart muscle behaves in a way that makes it more able to survive the loss of its blood supply during a heart attack.

Some evidence suggests that metformin might also be protective against some cancers, including breast cancer. This may just be because lower blood sugars deprive tumors of the glucose they need to grow aggressively. But it may also be due to the fact that metformin also has the ability to lower our levels of sex hormones. It lowers both testosterone and estradiol, which is the form of estrogen that postmenopausal women take when they use HRT made with "bioidentical" hormones. Estrogen stimulates several kinds of cancers, especially breast cancer.

This effect on hormones may also play a part in how metformin protects against heart attack, since high testosterone levels are associated with a higher risk of having one. Metformin lowers testosterone levels so well that it is prescribed to women with polycystic ovary syndrome, who have very high testosterone levels that lead them to experience facial hair growth and infertility. I have heard from women with PCOS who have taken metformin who complained that while it lowered their very high insulin resistance and even made them become fertile, their husbands really missed the effects of their earlier high testosterone levels. But this may mean that people who take metformin to control their diabetes may also experience a drop in hormones they would prefer to keep at their previous levels.

Is Plain Metformin Better Than Metformin ER?

Plain metformin is taken three times a day before meals. It has a stronger effect on the blood sugars that follow that meal, but it is also harder on your digestive tract than the extended release form of the drug. Since much of the effect of metformin occurs after it builds up in your body over a few days, it's likely that the impact of the extended release version is very similar over time.

The regular form also requires you to remember to take it at each meal. The once a day extended release version is easier to remember.

What Is the Right Dose of Metformin?

The right dose of any medication is something you can often only figure out by trial and error. Your doctor usually will start out prescribing a very low dose of metformin, usually 500 mg a day. Once you have gotten used to it and your digestive system has gone back to normal, doctors are supposed to raise the dose in 500 mg increments until you see a significant improvement in your blood sugars.

Most people won't see any substantial blood sugar lowering effect until they are taking 1000 mg a day. Many need at least 1500 mg to experience any effect.

But people frequently email me whose doctors have prescribed that low starting 500 mg dose and then never raised it. Not surprisingly, they report that metformin doesn't seem to work for them.

The highest dose that should be prescribed for regular metformin, the kind you take three times a day, is 2550 mg a day. For the Metformin ER (extended release) the maximum dose is 2000 mg a day. Some doctors get confused and prescribe the higher dose for the ER version. Mine did and it made me really sick until it wore off. So if you are feeling really toxic after taking your prescribed dose, check that you haven't been prescribed too much.

What Time of Day Should I Take Metformin ER?

With the extended release form of metformin, the tablet is designed so that it is supposed to release metformin steadily through the day. The drug is embedded in some kind of matrix that only lets a bit of metformin dissolve at a time. In some versions the used up matrix doesn't digest and may turn up in your toilet bowl looking like a white lump.

Though the original brand name version of the drug, Glucophage XR, reportedly releases the drug evenly throughout the whole 24 hours that the XR pill remains active, some of the cheaper generic versions use less effective matrices which release a lot of metformin over the first couple of hours and then less as the day goes by.

Some people find that because of this, they do best when they take their metformin before breakfast, so that drug's peak occurs during their lunch and dinner. However, this may make the drug slightly less effective at controlling their fasting blood sugars.

Some people divide their dose of the extended release form, since it is often prescribed in doses of several pills per day, and take one in the morning and one at night.

You'll only figure out what works best for you by careful experimentation. Just remember that you should *never* take more than your prescribed dose within a 24 hour period. If you want to move your daily dose from morning to evening you will have to skip a dose one morning and only take your metformin that evening. You should never take a day's worth of metformin in the morning and then take more later on in the same day.

Since metformin builds up in your body over a period lasting about a week, it takes a week or two until metformin gets up to full strength, and it keeps on working for up to a week when you stop taking it.

Is It Safe to Stop Taking Metformin?

My endocrinologist encouraged me to stop taking metformin at one point, to see if a symptom I was having was caused by the drug. Since then I have taken it for years at a stretch and then, periodically, gone on a "drug holiday," where I stopped taking it for a while. So unlike some other drugs, you can stop metformin without experiencing any dangerous rebound symptoms, though, of course, when you stop taking it your blood sugars will go back up.

Will I Ever Get over the Digestive Side Effects of Metformin?

Most people do get used to metformin after a week or two and don't even notice that they are taking it after that. Others never adjust. If your doctor started you on a dose higher than 500 mg a day and you are having trouble adapting, try lowering your dose for two weeks to see if that helps you adapt.

Most people find the extended release versions of metformin easier on their digestive system, though some brands of the extended release forms are much harder to tolerate than others. I can only tolerate the Teva brand, which Walgreens will dispense without any additional charge when I request it. Other pharmacies may only dispense whatever brand is cheapest. Try a couple of brands before you conclude you can't take handle it.

There is also a patented form, Glumetza, that some people report is much easier to tolerate when they can't tolerate the extended release form. The original branded version, Glucophage, also is reported to work much better for many people than the generics. If your insurance will cover it, it's worth asking your doctor to prescribe one of these.

Even when you feel like you have completely adapted to metformin, it can sometimes irritate the lower part of your esophagus and cause pain that can easily be mistaken for a heart attack. Needless to say, this can be scary.

I became familiar enough with that particular pain to ignore it, but only after my doctor did the tests to make sure my heart was fine. Taking your metformin after you've eaten a meal instead of on an empty stomach can help prevent this. If that doesn't work, heartburn pills usually calm it down, but I no longer recommend this solution, as taking drugs like Prilosec or Zantac for more than a brief period may raise your risk of dementia or some cancers.

It is also possible that this kind of pain is a sign you have a hiatal hernia. This is a common condition older people get that allows stomach acid to enter the esophagus because the valve that separates the esophagus from the stomach is no longer working properly.

Can Metformin Cause Hypos?

Metformin itself does not affect how much insulin your body secretes so it technically doesn't have the ability to cause hypos. However, because it limits liver dumping, it can worsen hypos caused by other drugs that do raise your insulin levels. This is even more true if you are eating a ketogenic diet. That's because ketogenic diets also limit your liver's ability to dump needed glucose into your blood when your blood sugars have dropped too low.

Sometimes people with Type 2 Diabetes who have just started taking metformin will find that they feel as if they are having a hypo, but when they test their blood sugar it will turn out it is nowhere near the range where true hypos occur—below 70 mg/dl {3.9}. This may happen because their blood sugars have been running very high and metformin lowers them enough to trigger the false hypo reaction we discussed on page 121.

I'm Not Responding to Metformin What Should I Do?

If you were diagnosed with a blood sugar level high enough to motivate your doctor to prescribe metformin right away, and if metformin doesn't seem to be lowering your blood sugar, it's possible you don't have classic Type 2 Diabetes but something else. One of the things you could have would be the adult-onset form of autoimmune diabetes very similar to Type 1 Diabetes, called LADA, as it is often misdiagnosed as Type 2 Diabetes when it strikes adults.

In that case, you need several tests to eliminate the possibility that your pancreas is suffering an autoimmune attack. One is the C-peptide test. This test will show if you are making the amounts of insulin characteristic of Type 2 Diabetes or the much lower amounts that point to developing autoimmune diabetes.

If there is any possibility you are developing the autoimmune form of diabetes, you should be tested for the antibodies used to diagnose Type 1 Diabetes. These are GAD or islet antibodies. Some family doctors are not familiar with these tests, so if you need them, you may have to make an appointment with an endocrinologist.

If the wait for the endocrinologist is lengthy, which it often is, since there aren't nearly enough endos to serve the population who need to see them, keep a close eye on your post-meal blood sugars. If they are rising from week to week, especially if they are above 300 mg/dl {22.2} even when you cut way down on the carbs you eat, call the endocrinologists office, tell the receptionist you are already scheduled for an appointment, and ask if you can speak to a nurse to make sure the rapid rise of your blood sugar isn't dangerous. Autoimmune diabetes can become an emergency pretty fast and you need to be screened for it to make sure that doesn't happen.

If you don't have autoimmune diabetes, your problem probably isn't insulin resistance but insulin deficiency. Repaglinide or insulin might be a better choice for you.

What's the Story on Repaglinide?

Repaglinide is a rarely prescribed drug that can be very useful. What it does is stimulate the beta cells in the pancreas to secrete insulin. There are older, less expensive drugs that also do this, which doctors frequently prescribe. These are the sulfonylurea drugs like glyburide, glimepiride, and glipizide.

The biggest problem with these older drugs is that they stimulate the pancreas for eight straight hours and sometimes longer. Insulin continually flows into your blood, which makes it very easy to hypo unless you eat a steady stream of carbs all day to prevent your blood sugar from going too low. People taking these drugs usually gain weight. These older insulin stimulating drugs also appear to stimulate a receptor in the heart in a way that raises your risk of having a heart attack.

Repaglinide also stimulates insulin release, but unlike the older drugs, robust research has shown that it does *not* raise the risk of having a heart attack. It also lasts a shorter time than do the sulfonylurea drugs. It only stimulates insulin secretion for about three hours, which makes it perfect for covering meals.

Repaglinide won't work unless you still have a significant number of beta cells left. Some people get diabetes because those cells, though they remain alive and healthy, aren't responding properly to the signals that tell a normal beta cell that blood sugar levels are rising so it's time to get working on pumping out the insulin. Repaglinide and the older sulfonylurea drugs stimulate these cells in a way that bypasses many steps involved in normal signaling. This can result in these drugs stimulating beta cells to produce surprising amounts of insulin.

The issue with all insulin stimulating pills, though, is that it takes a lot of experimentation to figure out how to match the amount of insulin the drug causes to be secreted to the precise amount of carbohydrate in your meal. So unless you get the dosing just right, repaglinide may also cause the roller-coaster blood sugars that lead to hunger and weight gain, though nowhere near as much as the older, longer lasting insulin-stimulating drugs do.

The other major issue with repaglinide, which is why I had to eventually stop taking it, is that when it is taken along with metformin, it may build up in your system and end up lasting much longer and lowering your blood sugar more aggressively than it does when taken alone. For some people with very high blood sugars, this extended, much stronger effect is a plus. The drug's label presents it that way. But for people whose blood sugars are closer to normal, that extra-long activity period can lead to nasty hypos.

When you are controlling your blood sugar using a carb-restricted diet, repaglinide can be helpful if used every now and. then. It can allow you to have an occasional carb up while still maintaining healthy blood sugar levels. For people who can get it working, it may make it possible to eat as much as one higher carbohydrate meal a day. But keep in mind if you use it this way that you will need to eat a lot less fat than would be healthy if you were eating a diet much lower in carbohydrate.

If you try repaglinide, your doctor should start you off on a very low dose, see how you respond, and only increase the dose if you don't see results from that starting dose. Some of us have genes which make us much more sensitive to repaglinide than others. If you have one of these gene variants, one half or even one quarter of a 1 mg pill might be all you need to cover an extra 30 grams of carbohydrate. People with normal sensitivity to the drug will need a larger dose.

Don't Insulin Stimulating Drugs Burn out Your Pancreas?

Doctor Bernstein stated that they did, back in the first edition of his *Diabetes Solutions* book. However subsequent research has found that while it is true that using these drugs for a long time can make it seem like the pancreas has conked out, the insulin secreting cells aren't really dead. If you stop the drug for a little while, they will wake right up and start secreting again.

What really kills the insulin secreting cells of many people who take these drugs are the high blood sugars they experience over the years they take them. Insulin stimulating drugs alone can't normalize the blood sugars of most people with Type 2 Diabetes who eat "normally." So the high blood sugars people experience while taking these drugs eventually leave them with dead, burnt out pancreases.

Using an insulin stimulating drug in a way that gives you post-meal blood sugars that stay below 140 mg/dl {7.8} or only spike above that level for an hour should be safe.

When Do I Need Insulin?

In an ideal world, you would be prescribed fast-acting insulin for use at mealtimes as soon as you were diagnosed with Type 2 Diabetes. Research has shown that using insulin to lower very high post-meal blood sugars for just a few months can provide a healing "beta cell rest" that will leave you with much better blood sugars for years to come, long after you have stopped taking the insulin. Unfortunately, the chances that your doctor will give you the three month's worth of insulin treatment this entails are zero.

The ADA's practice guidelines tell doctors not to prescribe insulin until every other possible drug has been tried, including the very expensive new ones whose dangerous side effects have yet to be discovered. (I did mention that the ADA is heavily funded by drug company donations, didn't I?) The ADA practice guidelines are echoed by the guidelines used by the World Health Organization and lots of other national health authorities. So right now, there isn't a place in the world I'm aware of where doctors prescribe fast-acting mealtime insulin to people newly diagnosed with Type 2 Diabetes, as helpful as it would be.

Doctors are also reluctant to prescribe insulin because the very thought of injecting themselves sends most of their patients into a panic. They prefer to prescribe pills as long as possible, too, because patients need a lot more education to be able to use insulin safely than they need when taking pills. Insulin can cause dangerous hypos, and using it correctly requires a certain amount of intelligence, which, sadly, not everybody has.

Another issue that keeps doctors from prescribing insulin to someone with Type 2 Diabetes is the widespread belief that using insulin always leads to weight gain, which will worsen existing control. This doesn't have to be true, especially if people aren't eating the very high carbohydrate meals so many people with diabetes are instructed to eat. Combining insulin with a lower carb intake—not necessarily a very low carb intake—can usually prevent weight gain, but doctors don't know this.

So with all this in mind, you can see that if a doctor tells you that you really need to start taking insulin, you really do, because they usually only tell you this years after insulin would have begun to be helpful.

If you are prescribed insulin, it will usually be what is called "basal insulin," which you take once a day. It only lowers your fasting blood sugar. You will still have to watch your carbs carefully to avoid a blood sugar spike after meals.

If you are recently diagnosed and can't get your blood sugar to drop below 250 mg/dl {11.1} after a "normal" high carb meal, even with metformin and a basal insulin, you should ask your doctor if you can try a short course of fast-acting insulin at mealtimes. This will usually require a referral to an endocrinologist.

Because I get a lot of emails from people who have read my other writings about the benefits of insulin, I want to reinforce one point made above. You shouldn't even think about trying fast-acting insulin unless the meals you plan to use it for would otherwise send your blood sugar soaring above 250 mg/dl {11.1}.

Using insulin when your blood sugar is closer to normal is much too risky. No matter how smart you are, you are likely to end up with serious hypos. Every person with Type 2 Diabetes who ends up in the ER with a hypo reduces their doctor's willingness to prescribe insulin to patients who could really use it and encourages doctors to maintain those patients on the expensive, potentially dangerous drugs that can't bring their blood sugars back down to the levels that prevent complications the way insulin can.

Does Starting Insulin Mean I Will Always Have to Take Insulin?

This is a common belief but it is absolutely not true. It goes along with another common belief, that going on insulin means you are so sick it's only a matter of time until you go blind, lose a foot, or die of a stroke.

The beliefs are common because a lot of people have seen their parents' generation suffer from diabetes back in the bad old days, which are as recent as 1991. Before then, when it wasn't common for people with diabetes to have access to home blood sugar testing, doctors put off prescribing insulin for people with Type 2 Diabetes as long as they could, since it is incredibly hard to avoid having hypos when you are injecting insulin with no idea of what your blood sugar might be.

So by the time someone diagnosed in the 1980s or earlier, was put on insulin, their A1C might have been as high as 11.0% for many years, Those years of exposure to very high blood sugars would have killed off their beta cells, and the high blood sugars that had produced those sky high A1Cs would have left their bodies riddled with heart disease and the classic diabetic complications. Even when they were given insulin, the belief that it was better for patients to maintain A1Cs of 9% or higher to avoid having hypos meant that most people who were using insulin had very high blood sugars all of the time.

It wasn't until 1992 that a very large research study of people with Type 1 diabetes called the DCCT discovered that lowering A1Cs to

7.0% — which was considered very low at the time — greatly lowered the incidence of diabetic blindness and kidney failure. A few years later, a study in a large group of people with Type 2 Diabetes, called the UKPDS, confirmed that they too benefited from achieving that lower A1C.

At the same time blood sugar meters became widely available for patients' use and metformin and faster, more effective, analog insulins hit the market. This made it possible for the first time for patients to aim for lower blood sugars safely. But it has taken another 20 years for a new generation of doctors to replace those trained in the '70s and '80s, who often continued to take a more relaxed attitude towards letting their patients run much higher blood sugars.

With that in mind you can understand why it wasn't unusual in the 1980s or even the 1990s, for someone to go on insulin shortly before they died, thanks to the havoc that had been wreaked on their bodies by years of extremely poor control. But that is no longer the case. Or at least it isn't if your family doctor is competent.

Nowadays, using insulin makes it more likely, not less, that you will be able to maintain the kind of good control that will prevent you from dying of anything caused by your diabetes. Not only that, but insulin is not in any way habit forming. You can start it and then stop it a few months later and go back to oral drugs or dietary control.

Help! I'm Terrified of Needles

Most people are scared of needles. This is because the needles we've encountered at the doctor's office when we've had to get immunizations hurt. So do the needles used to draw blood.

But guess what! Insulin needles are much thinner and shorter than those railroad spikes they use for immunizations and blood tests. They are so thin that if you have been prescribed the correct size, you shouldn't even feel it when an insulin needle pierces your skin.

Not only are insulin needles as thin as hairs, but when you inject insulin you don't inject it into a muscle, which is what happens when you are immunized, or into a vein, as is done when your blood is drawn. You inject insulin just under the skin into the pad of fat on your belly or upper thigh. The faster you inject, the more painless it is.

Dr. Bernstein suggests that when you first start injecting insulin, you hold a syringe or pen like a dart, about four or five inches away from where you plan to inject and then thrust it at your target as if you were throwing a dart. That approach is very helpful the first few times you give yourself an injection. But after a few tries most of us relax, because we learn it is actually a lot less painful to inject insulin than it is to pierce our fingers when we test our blood sugars.

Sometimes doctors, especially family doctors who were trained a long time ago, prescribe the much thicker, longer needles that were commonly used decades ago. These can hurt. The current advice is that you shouldn't need a needle longer than 6 millimeters, no matter how fat you might be, because a shorter needle makes it much less likely you will inject your insulin into a muscle. Doing that makes your insulin act too quickly and can cause serious hypos.

Most people do well with the ultra thin 31 or 32 gauge needles, which are the ones that are the thinnest. This prescribing advice is different from what doctors were taught even in the mid 2000s when I started using insulin, so some doctors still believe that if you have deep fat reserves you need a much longer needle. You don't.

If you get an insulin prescription, your doctor will also have to give you a prescription for needles. While you are at your appointment, be sure to ask your doctor what length and gauge they are prescribing. The higher the gauge, the thinner the needle. If you are prescribed 28 or 29 gauge needles, ask for the thinner, less painful 31 or 32 gauge.

What's the Best Way to Treat a Drug-Induced Hypo?

If you are using insulin or an insulin stimulating drug, a serious hypo is always a possibility. So when you are taking one of these drugs you should always keep some glucose with you in a pocket or in your purse. Always. You can buy glucose pills at the pharmacy or use candies that are made entirely of glucose like Smarties (the American kind) or the original, "classic," SweeTARTS. Glucose is labeled as "dextrose" on their labels, but they are the same thing. These candies have the advantage that if you run out you can get more at any convenience store or gas station that sells candy.

Carby foods that need to be digested are not a good source of glucose as digestion can be too slow to keep your hypo from getting much worse. Pure glucose goes right into your blood in less than 15 minutes, but carbs from food that needs to digest can take half an hour to an hour to get there.

If you suspect you are having a hypo while taking any of these drugs it's best to err on the side of overreacting rather than the opposite. If you have any concern that you might be heading for a hypo while taking insulin or an insulin-stimulating drug, test your blood sugar. If it's near 70 mg/dl {4.4}, take enough glucose to raise it 20 mg/dl {1.1}. The amount of glucose it will take depends on your size. The table we provided earlier in these pages is a good guide. You'll find it on Page 114. Test again in 15 minutes. If your blood sugar drops any lower than 70 mg/dl {4.4} take a larger dose of glucose and keep testing and taking glucose every fifteen minutes until you see your blood sugars rising again.

When you don't have your meter with you — and you should *always* have a meter with you if you are taking insulin or an insulin stimulating drug — if you think that you may be heading toward a hypo take some glucose right away. It's better to take too much and cause a high than to ignore a hypo and pass out.

If too much insulin or an insulin secreting drug are still working when your blood sugar is low, it can take surprisingly large doses of glucose to push your blood sugar up out of the danger zone. In an emergency a sugary soft drink or a glass of orange juice is a good way to get a lot of glucose into your system.

If you can't get your blood sugar to start climbing again when it is really low, call an ambulance.

What Can I Do to Avoid Having a Hypo?

Most people with Type 2 Diabetes are prescribed basal insulin, which will only lower their fasting blood sugar. These basal insulins rarely cause hypos unless you use too much or inject them into a blood vessel or muscle. Basal insulin is released very slowly, so you shouldn't expect it to eliminate the spikes caused by eating meals full of carbs. But this means it can be safely used along with carb-restricted diets.

It is beyond the scope of this book to explain to you how to use insulin. So I will say only that the best way to avoid hypos is to start out very cautiously with insulin or a drug like repaglinide that stimulates insulin release. Use a dose so small that it does absolutely nothing and then very slowly increase that dose, testing your blood sugar both when you are fasting and after meals until you get a good idea of how the drug affects you.

I always recommend that people who are going to be using insulin read the relevant chapters in the book, *Dr. Bernstein's Diabetes Solution,* several times, until the principles he explains have sunk in. This can be very helpful, especially if your doctor doesn't provide any real education in how to use it.

People with experience using insulin may be able, over time, to fine tune their doses to where they can get completely normal results. But if you are just starting out with insulin or an insulin stimulating drug, you simply don't have the experience and skill needed to do this. So don't try to lower your blood sugars with insulin below 95 mg/dl {5.3} and you will be much less likely to have hypos.

If you start seeing your blood sugar drop below 80 mg/dl {4.4} while using insulin or an insulin stimulating drug, when you are using the same dose you have been using for a while, you must cut your dose of the drug. While lower blood sugar levels are safe when achieved entirely through diet, when they are achieved with insulin you run the risk of losing the counterregulatory reaction that prevents you from having a severe hypo when your blood sugars start drifting down to this level. (This was explained on Page 139.)

Does Taking Insulin Raise the Risk of Cancer?

Because insulin is considered a growth hormone, this is a common belief, but it has not stood up to careful scrutiny by medical researchers. Cells don't appear to become cancerous because they are exposed to insulin.

What does happen is that cancer cells that have started growing for some other reason like an error in cell reproduction or a toxic exposure will grow faster in an environment loaded with their favorite food—blood glucose. They are also more likely to grow when the immune system has been damaged by long exposure to high blood sugars. So people whose diabetes has been bad enough to motivate their doctors to prescribe insulin do tend to get more cancers than people not using the drug. But it's their many years of exposure to high blood sugars that's at fault here, not the insulin they take.

So with that in mind, if you are afraid of cancer you should embrace insulin because of its superior ability to lower blood sugar and deprive cancer cells of their favorite food.

If you are worried about cancer, you should also avoid taking any of the incretin drugs like Januvia and Onglyza as this family of drugs works to lower blood sugar by turning off a gene that the immune system uses to destroy cells that have begun to metastasize into melanoma, prostate, and ovarian cancer cells. While these drugs don't appear to cause these cancers, they turn off genes in a way that may promote their growth if there are already any of these kinds of cancer cells in your body.

Some very high quality research that the drug companies have attempted, unsuccessfully to dismiss, suggests that Januvia and the injected incretin drugs, Byetta, Bydureon, and Victoza (a.k.a. Saxenda) also cause abnormal growths to develop in the pancreas. These are a type that over time turns into tumors. They are also impossible to detect with any technology currently in general use. The research that detected them involved doing autopsies on people who had been taking these drugs after they had died of something else. You can't detect them in a living person, as these growths can only be seen when you cut into the pancreas, which will severely damage it. They go undetected until you get the symptoms of pancreatic cancer—a cancer that is almost always fatal once those symptoms have appeared.

Victoza is also associated with tumors of the thyroid.

The drug companies have put a lot of effort into assuring doctors they shouldn't worry about the research that found these precancerous growths in the pancreases of people who had been taking these drugs. That's because the drugs that appear to cause them are among the most profitable drugs in the world. But the studies I've carefully reviewed suggest that it will be another decade until the truth is evident—and if these abnormal growths do turn out to cause fatal pancreatic cancers, a lot of people with Type 2 Diabetes are going to be dying, tragically and completely unnecessarily.

You can learn more about the research on which these claims are made on the web pages "DPP-4 Inhibitors Januvia, Onglyza, Trajenta, Combiglyze, Janumet, and Jentadueto," which you'll find at **http://www.bloodsugar101.com/18538604.php** and" GLP-1 Agonists: Byetta, Adlixin, Victoza, Saxenda, Bydureon, Trulicity, Tanzeum," found at **http://www.bloodsugar101.com/18538438.ph**p.

Why isn't Insulin Lowering My Blood Sugar to Near Normal?

Family doctors hate prescribing insulin because finding the right dose for a patient is complicated. Two patients of the same age and size, with the same Type 2 Diabetes diagnosis, may need very different doses. But doctors don't have time to dial in doses exactly, so they are happy to get close and declare victory. Not only that, but "close" is always a lot less than the amount that would provide truly normal blood sugars because of the fear of hypos. It's safer to give the patient a low dose that gives them a little better control with very small chance of them ending up in the ER than to prescribe the a higher dose that used properly might provide extremely good blood sugars.

Once you are prescribed insulin, no one will be looking over your shoulder to see how you use it. So if you are a moderately intelligent person who is willing to do some studying, you can often tweak your insulin dose on your own and find the sweet spot that gives you much better control while still keeping you safe.

How you do that is beyond the scope of this book. You can learn much more on that topic from books by experts like *Dr. Bernstein's Diabetes Solution, Think Like A Pancreas*, by Gary Scheiner, and John Walsh's *Using Insulin*.

If you do decide to tweak your dose, be extremely cautious. Make very small changes and use your meter to make sure you are not risking hypos.

What's the Difference Between Insulin Pens and Needles?

There are two ways to inject insulin. One is to use a syringe with units marked on its side. This requires that you draw up the correct-sized dose from a glass vial. It's a bit tricky getting just the right dose with a syringe.

The other way you inject insulin is with an insulin pen. This is a device that is designed to look like, you guessed it, a pen, but is really a small vial of insulin with some fancy engineering that lets you select exactly how many units you want to inject. Unlike a syringe, the pen is reusable until the insulin runs out. Pens use screw-on pen needles for which you need a separate prescription.

Pens are far more convenient than syringes and make it much less likely you will get the wrong dose. They also have the advantage that you aren't as likely to ruin a whole bottle's worth of insulin by continually piercing it with syringes that may introduce contaminants into the vial or by exposing it to temperatures that are damagingly high or low. Either can "kill" your insulin or make it lose its potency. When you use pens, if you screw up and leave your diabetes kit in a hot car, you will still have more pens left in the fridge, as several pens will be dispensed with your monthly prescription.

But pens are more expensive than vials and syringes, so some cheapskate insurance plans won't cover them unless your doctor writes them a letter stating that you are having trouble using a vial accurately due to visual problems, arthritic hands, or increasing age.

The other problem with pens is that you will have to waste some insulin every time you use your pen, because you have to squirt a little insulin before you inject, to prime the pen. If you use mealtime insulin, you may end up having to have your doctor order more units of insulin for you when prescribing pens than they would when prescribing needles.

The older, cheap regular human insulins may not be available in pens, depending on what country you live in. But since most people use these older, slower insulins because they can't afford more expensive ones, the extra price they'd have to pay to get their insulin in a pen would probably keep them from buying them, anyway.

Some of the very newest basal insulins only come in pens. That is because the amount of insulin found in each drop of these new insulins is much higher than that of the insulins you can use with a syringe. So one unit of the new insulin contains two or three more times as much actual insulin than a unit of the older stuff does. To prevent people overdosing, the company does not sell a vial version. Using a highly concentrated vial insulin would require that you use specially marked syringes.

What Is the Best Basal Insulin?

There are several different brands of expensive, patented basal insulin on the market now, including several new ones introduced since 2016. Among the newest are some very long-lasting ones and some that come in highly concentrated versions specially formulated for people who need to take very large doses. These branded basal insulins include Lantus, Levemir, Tresiba, and Toujeo. They each differ in how long they remain active in the body, with Levemir lasting the shortest time and Tresiba the longest. A generic form of Lantus is also available called Basaglar.

For people with poor or no insurance coverage or older people hitting the Medicare "donut hole" who can't afford the many hundreds of dollars a month these branded insulins cost, there are two mediocre but much, much cheaper regular human insulins available that can be used to replace the more expensive, longer lasting basals. These cheaper insulins are, Novolin N or Humulin N. The N stands for "NPH."

These NPH insulins are better than nothing but they are much harder to use to get tight control. They don't release insulin into your system slowly and steadily the way the newer, more expensive versions do. Instead they tend to be absorbed in a way where the insulin level slowly rises to a peak and then drops down again, with that peak occurring at unpredictable times. Because they are not very long-lasting, you may have to inject one of these insulins two or three times a day to get full 24 hour coverage. If you switch to one of these cheap NPH insulins from a branded version, your doctor will have to tell you which dose to use as the dose may not be equivalent to what you were taking.

Walmart sells the N insulins under the Relion brand name for a price much cheaper than most other drug stores. CVS may too. Call several different pharmacies to make sure you pay the lowest price.

Basaglar is a biosimilar version of insulin glargine, the insulin found in Lantus, the bestselling long-lasting basal insulin. Though it is, basically, a generic version of Lantus, which has now gone off patent, you will need a new prescription from your doctor to get it. Pharmacists can't dispense it instead of the brand name Lantus the way they could if this biosimilar was treated as a generic. Basaglar only comes in pens.

Since it is priced 15% lower than Lantus, it is likely that some insurers will force the people with Type 2 Diabetes to use Basaglar rather than one of the more expensive patented basal insulins. Though it is cheaper than Lantus, this biosimilar is still around 12 times more expensive than the NPH insulin you can buy at Walmart.

I have heard reports from Europe that Basaglar does not work as well as actual Lantus. If you are forced to switch and can't get it working, ask your doctor to write to your insurance company explaining why you need to go back on the Lantus that used to work so well for you. Some insurers will cover a drug that is not on their formulary if your doctor can make a strong case for why you need it.

When people use the large doses usually prescribed for insulin resistant people with Type 2 Diabetes, most of the basal insulins usually last for 24 hours or longer. However, if you use a small dose—one closer to 20 units than 100, it may last for a shorter time and leave you with a period each day when your fasting blood sugar is too high. The solution to this can be to split your dose and take half of it in the morning and half before bed.

Alternatively, if your insurance covers it, you can switch to the newer basal insulin, Tresiba, which users report lasts longer and works very well. It and some other newer basal insulins come in different versions that are more concentrated than standard insulin is, Because the concentration is different you should never, ever, use a syringe to draw these high concentration insulins out of a pen. The units on the syringe won't match the units you are actually getting and you can have a severe hypo if you get this wrong.

If you have to use NPH due to financial considerations, read the book, "*Dr. Bernstein's Diabetes Solution,*" very carefully as Dr. Bernstein explains how to dose NPH in great detail.

I frequently hear from people who are as disgusted as I am at the way that insulin prices have tripled in the United States over the past eight years. This is entirely caused by drug company greed. The insulins whose prices tripled were old products that have been sold quite profitably for decades at much lower prices. Drug companies get away with this kind of price gouging because Congress continues to forbid Medicare and Medicaid to negotiate drug prices, unlike every other government health program in the world. Only Congress can fix this. So if this upsets you, contact your congresspeople and demand that the insulin cartel be forced to roll back these unjustifiable price increases.

Why Did I Suddenly Get a Huge Hypo Taking My Usual Dose of Lantus?

There are several possible explanations for why you might suddenly have a hypo while using your usual dose of a long-acting basal insulin. One is that you accidentally injected it into a muscle or blood vessel instead of a patch of fat.

What makes some insulins slow-acting is that they are engineered to resist absorption from your body fat, so that only a small amount is absorbed into your blood at any one time. But once these insulins get into your blood they act just like fast-acting insulins. So if you shoot a day's worth of Lantus into a vein, it can become a crisis that may require you to take a huge dose of glucose and then chug carbs for three or four hours more until this now-fast-acting insulin is used up. If your blood sugar doesn't stop dropping after you take the glucose and lots of carbs, an immediate trip to the ER may be the best solution.

But there are other reasons why you might have gotten way too much basal insulin. If you also use a fast-acting insulin, you may have absentmindedly grabbed the wrong pen or vial and injected a basal-sized dose of the fast-acting insulin instead of your basal. This happens more than you would expect. This too can quickly turn into an emergency.

One last possibility is that you may have spaced out and given yourself two shots of basal after having forgotten that you had already taken your daily shot. This is more likely to happen to people who are developing memory problems, but it can happen to anyone if they are distracted enough. That's why it's a good idea to get into the habit of making a note in a log every time you take your daily shot. Keep it handy, perhaps on your phone. Get into the habit of always checking your log before you inject, to be sure you don't inject twice.

What Is the Difference Between Humulin, Humalog, and Novolog?

These are all fast-acting insulins which are meant to be injected at mealtimes in doses that, ideally, are of the proper size to match the amount of carbohydrate in your meal.

Humulin R and Novolin R are the slowest of these mealtime insulins. They contain regular human insulin, which is an insulin whose molecule is identical to the insulin molecules your pancreas makes. However, when injected into your fat tissue, these human insulins absorb very slowly. They take at least an hour to start working and as long as five hours to finally stop. This can make them very tough to use if you are trying to cover high carbohydrate meals with them.

They do have the advantage of being cheap if you buy them at Walmart. They are usually much more expensive at other pharmacies. You can also buy these regular human insulins without a prescription in most places in the United States. However it may be impossible to buy the needles you need to use to inject them without a prescription.

Humalog, Novolog (called NovoRapid in the UK), and Apidra are branded, fast-acting, analog insulins that absorb faster after you inject them. They act more quickly than the regular human insulin we just described. What makes them faster is that one or two different amino acids have been inserted into their molecular structure replacing the ones found in the stuff your body makes. Despite these tiny differences from regular human insulin, once they reach your blood stream these analog insulins interact with the receptors in your cells the same way regular human insulin does.

Because each brand of analog insulin uses a different mechanism to make the insulin be absorbed more quickly, some start working faster than others or may take longer to leave the body. Apidra is the fastest, and the one most like the insulin your pancreas secretes in terms of how fast it acts, but very few insurers cover it. This is because the company that sells it could never figure out how to properly price and promote it, not because there is anything wrong with it.

There is a new insulin, Fiasp, which is supposed to be a faster version of Novolog. It has been available in Europe since the beginning of 2017 and is expected to be approved in the United States by the end of 2017.

Very few family doctors have the expertise or time to help you learn how to dose any of these fast-acting insulins properly and the family doctors who are willing to prescribe them for people with Type 2 Diabetes often use an old fashioned, very crude dosing formula, based entirely on what your blood sugar is before you take it, not on how many carbs you are going to eat. This makes the insulin far less effective than it would be had it been prescribed using more modern dosing methods.

If you are prescribed mealtime insulin and don't find that it is giving you post-meal numbers very close to normal, it is time to head to a very good endocrinologist and ask that they get you the same kind of training people with Type 1 Diabetes get when they use these insulins.

What is 70/30 Insulin?

The 70/30 insulins are mixtures of basal and fast-acting insulin. The appeal is that you only have to buy one vial or box of pens, not two. But since you can't adjust the doses separately, you usually can't get good meal-time coverage and good fasting coverage at the same time.

The fast-acting insulin in this mixture will only cover the meal immediately following the time you inject it, while the basal insulin will keep on working for hours. You can't inject more because you are likely to get too much basal.

A 70/30 insulin isn't likely to give you the kind of good control you need on its own and it can give you hypos at mealtime if you try to lower your carbs while taking it. Because 70/30 insulins were what people used to use back in the bad old days, there are still family doctors prescribing it.

What Dose of Insulin Should I Be Taking?

It is disturbing how often people email me with this question. They are paying their doctors to prescribe this potentially dangerous medication, so these doctors should have given them this answer. They also should also have made their patients aware of how carefully insulin needs to be dosed and how dangerous it could be to take advice about their insulin dosage from some stranger they meet on the Internet.

The amount of insulin that constitutes the proper dose is different from person to person. A doctor should be starting you out at a low dose and instructing you how to adjust that dose until you have achieved good control. No one who does not have access to your medical records should be telling you what dose to use. Not me, not some guy on some diabetes forum.

If you don't understand insulin dosing, you must contact the staff at your doctor's office and tell them you need more help. If the practice isn't able to supply that help, ask for a referral to an endocrinologist.

Don't ask your cousin who takes insulin what dose he takes and copy it. Your cousin might be twice as insulin resistant as you are and his dose could put you into a coma.

Don't mess around with doses based on what you read in even the very best books until you've worked with your doctor to get at least close to where you need to be.

Why Can't I Lower My Blood Sugar Even with a Huge Dose of Insulin?

There are several rare conditions that can make a person extremely insulin resistant, to the point where they can be injecting 300 units of insulin a day and still be seeing very high blood sugars.

Because these conditions are so rare, when doctors find you are running extremely high blood sugars after they have prescribed a huge dose of insulin, they may assume you aren't really taking your shots and are lying about it. This isn't because these doctors are paranoid or hate their patients. There *are* patients who do this, perhaps because they are terrified of needles and afraid to appear cowardly by admitting it.

But because patients lie, it can be really tough to get the treatment you need when you are not responding to doses of insulin that should be enough to knock out an elephant. If you find yourself in this situation, you need to get yourself to an endocrinologist—and not just any endocrinologist, but a truly expert one. You'll find them at major medical centers affiliated with medical schools. They can run the tests needed to diagnose and treat the unusual conditions you may be suffering from.

Why Won't My Doctor Prescribe the New Inhaled Insulin?

Afrezza is an inhaled, very fast-acting mealtime insulin that may well be an excellent product. But the company that brought it to market has always been run by people with no previous experience developing diabetes drugs or, in fact, any other pharmaceutical drugs. They did such a poor job designing the trials that were used to get Afrezza approved that any properly trained doctor who reads the drug's official prescribing information will conclude that it doesn't work and may harm your lungs.

Anecdotal information from a very small group of people who have been getting Afrezza to work for them, suggests that if you are patient and willing to experiment you may be able to get Afrezza to work very well at mealtimes. But the people who are getting it to work are almost all people with Type 1 Diabetes who use much, much smaller doses than people with Type 2 usually need. Unfortunately, Afrezza is very expensive and with the way Afrezza has been packaged, you may not be able to afford enough doses of it to make it work in place of injected fast-acting insulin, especially if you are an insulin resistant person with Type 2 Diabetes using the much larger doses that Type 2 people need.

If you do get a prescription for Afrezza, you need to be aware that it is extremely fast-acting. This means it hits your blood stream much faster than injected insulin and is out of your body much faster, too. If your digestion is slow, Afrezza may get into your blood before the carbs from your meal turn into blood glucose. This can cause hypos. Though there are investors posting in social media that Afrezza can't cause hypos, I have been contacted by users who reported that they had indeed experienced them.

If you are already using injected fast-acting insulin, you'll need to know that 12 units of Afrezza will lower your blood sugar a lot less than does 12 units of any of the injected fast-acting insulins, so you may need to use a lot more. You may also need a second dose an hour after you eat, because Afrezza finishes working so fast that there may still be too much glucose in your blood two hours after eating when it has finished working.

Why Does My Blood Pressure Go up When I Take Certain Diabetes Drugs?

Quite a few diabetes drugs cause insulin to be secreted. This includes drugs like Januvia, Onglyza, Bydureon, and Victoza. Some of us find that having more insulin in our bloodstreams, even when it is lowering our blood sugars, will push up our blood pressure. I am not sure why this is, but I have observed it happen myself a couple times.

Researchers have speculated that it may have something to do with how insulin affects our blood levels of sodium. Some research has found that after four months, blood pressures that originally rose when people started insulin dropped back to their original levels. This relationship between higher insulin levels and higher blood pressure might partially explain why so many people who lower their carbs, and thus the amount of insulin their bodies need to secrete, end up with lower blood pressures, too.

Why Do I Get Either Highs or Hypos with Mealtime Insulins?

Different people respond differently to the same brand of insulin. Some will do really well on a brand that another person finds either leaves them with undesirable highs or makes them hypo, with nothing in between.

In the past when people wrote to tell me that they were having a terrible time getting their fast-acting insulin to work, I'd suggest they ask their doctor to switch them to a different brand. But now that the insulin companies have pushed their prices up to obscene levels, the companies that make insulin are cutting deals with insurers where the insurer gets a big break on the price of one brand of insulin, as long as they don't prescribe the brands sold by their competitors. This may make it impossible to get your insurer to pay for a brand they have stopped covering, even though it might work much better for you.

If you are really having a tough time with an insulin your insurance has made you use, ask your doctor to write the insurer a letter explaining why you need to use a competing brand. If that doesn't work, change your insurance as soon as possible. If your insurance is provided by your employer, contact employee benefits and explain why the plan they have signed you up for is threatening to ruin your health.

And write to your congresspeople, pointing out that these sweetheart deals the drug companies are making with insurers are severely damaging the health of the people lawmakers are supposed to protect. Because they are.

I Can't Afford Insulin but I Need It What Do I Do?

Drug companies maintain what they call "Patient Assistance Programs" that supply their insulins either at a deep discount or for free to needy people who can't otherwise afford them. The best way to find these programs is to Google "Insulin patient assistance programs."

Unfortunately, many of these programs won't help you if you are on Medicare or Medicaid. If that's your situation, you may need to contact your local social service organization to learn if there are any state assistance programs that might help you.

Patient assistance programs may also not help you if you earn a comfortable middle class income but have chosen your insurance plan unwisely. If that is your situation, you may have to use the cheaper regular human insulins you can buy at Walmart or CVS for about $27 a vial and inject with a syringe, rather than the much more expensive branded insulins.

If you switch from using an expensive branded insulin to the cheap human insulins you may also have to work with your doctor to adjust the dose. Don't try doing this on your own unless you have a lot of experience with insulin dosing.

You must use a meter and test strips if you are using insulin. So if you can't afford prescription strips or don't have a prescription, tell registered pharmacist at Walmart that you are using insulin and ask them which of their inexpensive meters would be the most accurate for avoiding hypos. The models they sell keep changing so fast that it's impossible to rely on recommendations you read online as they may refer to outdated models.

If you have been resisting cutting your carbs until now, it's time to give it a try. Many people find that when they cut way down on how much carbohydrate they eat, their blood sugar comes down to where they don't need to use any insulin or can get by with using a lot less.

Reread the instructions you'll find in Chapter Three to learn how.

Why Am I Suddenly Having Hypos on Drugs That Used to Work Fine?

Many things can change the way that you respond to drugs that have hitherto worked for you. If a drug seems to have stopped working, it may be because you are losing more beta cells. If the drug is one that stimulates insulin secretion, you may just need to take a break, as these drugs can sometimes temporarily shut down your beta cells if you have been using them for a long time.

But sometimes drugs seem to become *more* effective, not less, after you have been taking them for a while. This can be especially true of insulin and drugs that stimulate insulin secretion. One cause might be that you have lowered your blood sugar enough to have eliminated the acquired insulin resistance that is a response to very high blood sugars. This would make you need less insulin to cover the same amount of carbohydrate.

If you suddenly start having hypos while taking insulin or an insulin stimulating drug, it is also possible that your digestive tract has stopped working properly. If your digestion has slowed, glucose may not be reaching your bloodstream until hours after it would normally. Then your insulin gets into your bloodstream before the glucose does which sends your blood sugar plummeting.

If you start seeing real hypos—blood sugars in the 60s or below {3.3 or lower}, stop taking the medication that has been causing them and see your doctor. Having more than one or two hypos can lead to your having another hypo that is much worse as you may lose your hypo awareness, which we discussed earlier on Page 139. When this happens, it isn't a gradual process. You can easily go from seeing 64 mg/dl {3.6} after a meal to seeing 40 mg/dl {2.2} without seeing any readings in-between. Once you have one hypo in the 40s you are likely to see even lower hypos that can become life threatening.

So report frequent hypos to your doctor and, if possible, get an appointment with an endocrinologist who will have much more experience with helping patients work out the right doses of the insulins they take.

Victoza, Januvia, and/or Jardiance Work Great Why Do You Scare People Away from Taking Them?

I don't ever suggest that these drugs don't lower blood sugar. They do. Sometimes very well. The problem is that the way they lower blood sugar has unintended consequences throughout your body, because the genes they mess with do many other things besides regulating blood sugar. Because of the way the drug approval process works, none of these other things have been adequately investigated. Over the years, I have seen several heavily prescribed diabetes drugs turn out to have very serious side effects that only were made public when their patents had almost expired. I suspect to see the same thing happen with these new drugs, too.

I warned readers of my blog about the severe side effects of Avandia almost a year before the news was made public that it increased the risk of having a heart attack. I also warned readers that Avandia and the other similar drug in the same class, Actos, caused irreversible osteoporosis that could lead to broken bones in older people. Now these drugs are far less frequently prescribed.

The most worrisome side effects of the newest drugs involve cancer, and not just any cancer but some of the most fatal cancers: pancreatic cancer and melanoma. I see no reason to gamble that the evidence pointing to this possibility is any less likely to prove out than the evidence I found for Avandia and Actos. So I would wait, at a minimum, until the patent for the first of the incretin drugs, Januvia, expires in 2022 before taking an incretin drug.

The SGLT-2 drugs are so new that the patent for the first of them, Invokana, won't expire until 2029. It is only when the patents for billion-dollar profit generating drugs expire and they get replaced by cheaper generics that researchers find the courage to publish the studies that deal them death blows. Unfortunately, by that time, a lot of people who have been taking them for the 14 years since they were approved will have developed their potentially life-altering side effects.

You can read about the specific problems identified with these newer drugs on these web pages: "SGLT2 Inhibitors, Farxiga, Invokana, Jardiance. Questionable New Drugs," which you'll find at **http://www.bloodsugar101.com/36474059.php**, "DPP-4 Inhibitors Januvia, Onglyza, Trajenta, Combiglyze, Janumet, and Jentadueto" found at **http://www.bloodsugar101.com/18538604.php** and "GLP-1 Agonists: Byetta, Adlixin, Victoza, Saxenda, Bydureon, Trulicity, Tanzeum," found at **http://www.bloodsugar101.com/18538438.php**.

Doesn't Jardiance Prevent Heart Attacks?

This is what the drug reps have told family doctors. It isn't a complete lie but it definitely stretches the truth. The research study this claim is based on found that people who already had had heart attacks or stents had slightly fewer heart attacks going forward when taking Jardiance, but they had more strokes. Others who took the drug who had not already been diagnosed with significant heart disease didn't see a significant preventive effect. Some of them had more strokes.

Most importantly, the same study showed the drug did a very poor job of lowering blood sugar in most of those who took it. After taking Jardiance for four years the drug only lowered subjects' A1C an average 0.24% when taken at a low dose and 0.36% when taken at its highest dose. Its benefit to those with a history of previous heart attacks may have been due to the diuretic effect of the drug. You can read the specifics about the way that the drug company has stretched the truth about this drug on the Blood Sugar 101 web page, "SGLT2 Inhibitors, Farxiga, Invokana, Jardiance. Questionable New Drugs," found at **http://www.phlaunt.com/diabetes/36474059.php**.

Makers of several competing drugs in the same family are working diligently on studies they hope will show the same benefit for their drugs. Some epidemiological data is being used to suggest that Farxiga helps prevent heart failure, which is what diuretics do—i.e. water pills. The chances are that a more detailed study will find that all drugs in this class have the effects you would expect to see from a good diuretic but that their effect on blood sugar is not strong enough to justify risking their other side effects.

And these side effects are troubling. The FDA has warned that all drugs in this class can increase the likelihood of toe amputations and can also cause people with Type 2 Diabetes to develop diabetic keto-acidosis. This last issue suggests that no one who is eating a ketogenic diet should take Invokana, Farxiga, or Jardiance which all have the same effect, as the rising ketone levels in the blood may become toxic if the drug stops the kidneys from properly eliminating ketones.

How Can I Check on the Safety of a New Drug My Doctor Prescribes?

The best way to learn about any new drug is to download a copy of the drug's official label. You can find it by Googling the name of the drug followed by the words, "prescribing information." There is usually a patient's version and a doctor's version of this label. The patient's version is dumbed down and lists only what the FDA considers the most significant side effects of the drug. The physician's version will go into depth about how the drug works, what other drugs it may interact with, what severe and milder side effects it may cause, and how it should be dosed. The physician's version of the prescribing information will also tell you how effective the drug really is.

Reading the physician's version of the prescribing information may be very tough, as parts are written in what can be very baffling medical terminology. But when you look up these terms, most turn out to just be a word that makes something simple sound complex. "Hyper-glycemia," is just our old friend high blood sugar. "Urticaria," is hives. Edema is watery swelling. Once you learn a couple of these words, the prescribing information is much easier to understand and you can learn a great deal about what a drug does and does not do.

The label is also where you will learn that most of the expensive drugs your doctor may suggest only lower A1C, on average, by .5%. It is also where you will learn that when you take an expensive new drug along with metformin, the combined effect of the two drugs may be no greater than that of plain metformin alone.

One problem with the prescribing information is that it will include a long list of the side effects that occurred in 2% or less of the people who took it. This list does not distinguish between side effects that were mild and transient and those that were permanent and life-altering.

Doctors rarely know any more than you do about which side effects on that long list are a serious concern. Two percent sounds like a small number, but if ten million people are taking the drug and two percent got the side effect that means two hundred thousand people experienced it. If that side effect turns out to be something serious, like permanent damage to joints or tinnitus, that's a lot of people whose lives may have been ruined unnecessarily.

So if you are having a new, concerning symptom while taking a new drug and that symptom appears on the list, it is a very good idea to stop taking it. Just make sure before you stop taking any drug that it isn't one of a small number of drugs where stopping it abruptly can cause dangerous rebound effects. Your pharmacist can tell you if this would be the case.

After a drug is approved, the FDA makes companies update their labels with information about new side effects as they are reported. But busy family doctors don't have the time to keep up with all the new information that comes out about each of the dozens of drugs they routinely prescribe. So don't expect them to be aware of new problems with drugs you are taking. But *you* need to be because you are the person who may be harmed by one.

If what you read in a drug's prescribing information is too befuddling, call the registered pharmacist who works for the pharmacy that dispenses your drugs. This is not the clerk who hands you your prescription but someone with a specialized degree who is paid a high salary to make sure that the pharmacy doesn't kill anyone by accident. Ask your pharmacist about any potential drug interactions or side effects that concern you.

Help! I Read That a Drug I Take Can Cause Diabetes

Several classes of very commonly prescribed drugs appear to significantly raise the risk that a person will develop diabetes. As just explained, drug companies generally keep this information hidden until their blockbuster drugs' patents expire, so we have only recently learned that the statin drugs, as a class, have this effect.

SSRI antidepressants like Prozac have also been shown to significantly increase the likelihood that people who take them will develop Type 2 Diabetes. Drug companies argued for years that this was because people who go on to develop diabetes are more depressive and hence more likely to take their drugs. But some good work by some researchers who were not on drug company payrolls found that a control group of people with depression who did not take antidepressants did *not* go on to develop diabetes anywhere near as frequently as did the people who took the antidepressant drugs. It isn't clear whether these drugs damage blood sugar control because of the way they remodel structures in the brain or because they promote weight gain and increased insulin resistance.

The thiazide diuretics prescribed for lowering blood pressure also appear to raise the risk of diabetes. These drugs flush potassium out of our blood streams. But it turns out that potassium plays a vital role in the secretion of insulin and in the process by which insulin helps cells take in glucose. It is believed these drugs are less likely to worsen your blood sugar if you take extra potassium to counteract the loss these drugs can cause. But talk to your registered pharmacist before you start taking extra potassium. There are other drugs you might be taking that make it dangerous to supplement with this element. The thiazide diuretics may also raise blood sugar just because they decrease the amount of fluid in the blood stream, which increases the concentration of glucose.

If your blood sugar is well controlled while you are taking one of these thiazide drugs there is no reason to stop taking it. They work very well to control high blood pressure, and blood pressure control is almost as important for people with diabetes as blood sugar control.

Beta blockers are another family of drugs that appear to raise the risk of developing diabetes. Their main function is to keep your body from secreting the stress hormones that increase insulin resistance and make the liver dump glucose. But it turns out they also may limit the ability of the beta cells to secrete insulin. Supposedly the beta-1 selective beta blockers like atenolol are less likely to have this effect.

By the way, you should never let a doctor prescribe you a beta blocker if you are taking insulin or one of the oral drugs that force your body to secrete insulin. That's because beta blockers block the stress hormones that normally raise your blood sugar when it starts to go dangerously low. So beta blockers can make it much easier to have a severe hypo. Other blood pressure drugs are a better choice for people with diabetes who take insulin stimulating drugs or insulin.

Should I Stop Taking This Drug That Worsens Blood Sugar?

Because several of the drugs that can worsen your blood sugar are habit forming and can cause severe side effects if stopped suddenly, you should not stop taking them until you talk with your doctor or a pharmacist about whether it would be safe to do so.

Beta blockers and SSRI antidepressants are drugs that can cause severe problems if you stop them suddenly. Stopping beta blockers abruptly can result in your having a heart attack as the stress hormones you have turned off come roaring back. Stopping SSRI antidepressants can cause severe withdrawal symptoms that go way beyond a return of depression. Some other blood pressure drugs cause rebound very high blood pressures. So before you stop taking any drug you have been taking for a while, make certain it is safe to do so.

Before you make the decision to stop a useful drug, it's also worth considering the extent to which it raises your blood sugar. If it is only by a small amount that doesn't make it impossible for you to keep your blood sugars in a range low enough to prevent complications, it may be worth staying on the drug and eating a bit less carbohydrate to limit its effects.

Should I Stop Taking a Statin?

There is an almost fanatical cult online of people who demonize statins. This makes sense, as there is also a fanatical cult of doctors who think everyone over the age of 30, along with their pets and, perhaps, their potted plants, should be taking a statin.

So when you venture to answer the question, "Should I stop taking a statin" you will hear from people who have very strong opinions both pro and con—opinions about which they can get very emotional.

My take on this, based on the research I've reviewed, is that statins can be helpful if you have had a heart attack in the past or have had a stent inserted, especially if you are a middle aged man. Likewise, if a blood test found that you have a high level of cardiac-specific C-reactive protein in your blood, a statin might indeed help prevent a heart attack. Cardiac specific C-reactive protein is a substance that, when it is high, suggests you have a lot of inflammation in your arteries. Don't confuse it with C-peptide, which is a completely different substance that is a byproduct of insulin synthesis.

Statins do a good job of fighting inflammation in your arteries. This appears to be why they do seem to help prevent some people from having heart attacks, rather than the fact that they also lower LDL cholesterol. If you are currently taking a statin and having no problems, you are probably safer continuing to take it.

I would never suggest, as do too many cultish anti-statinators, that someone should immediately stop taking a statin just because they have cut back on their carbs. It takes years of maintaining excellent blood sugar control to undo the damage caused by years of feasting on high carb sugary treats laced with heart-damaging trans fat. If you have had undiagnosed high blood sugars for years, it's possible you have significant amounts of both plaque and inflammation in your arteries. If so, a statin might be exactly what you need to prevent inflammation from leading to the ruptured plaques that lead to heart attacks.

If you don't know what to think, it might be useful to get a coronary calcium scan. These cost about $99 and are not usually covered by insurance. You can usually get this test without needing a doctor's referral. It will show how much calcium has been deposited in your coronary arteries. A low score should be reassuring that the arteries serving your heart are in pretty good shape. A higher score might make you reconsider refusing a statin.

Will a Cortisone Drug Permanently Raise My Blood Sugar?

Corticosteroids like prednisone can dramatically worsen your blood sugar when taken internally, though cortisone creams are less likely to have this effect. Doctors will assure you that this effect is temporary, but my own experience with a course of prednisone that raised my prediabetic blood sugars a good 100 mg/dl {5.1} was that "temporary" lasted for about fourteen years. I have heard from other people who also found that a single course of prednisone permanently raised their blood sugars from a mildly diabetic level, which had been easy to manage with diet, to one that was much more severe.

There are serious conditions for which you really need to take corticosteroids. These are usually autoimmune inflammatory conditions where without the corticosteroid your body and or brain may suffer devastating, permanent injury. If that's why your doctor prescribed a corticosteroid, you will have to take it and accept that your blood sugar is going to be very high for a while and possibly even for a very long while. That said, most people with diabetes do see their blood sugar drop back to their previous levels when the corticosteroid treatment is finished.

The real problem with these drugs is that too many doctors use cortisone injections as a placebo—a handy way to make patients feel like they got something for their money after visiting a doctor for back pain or an aching knee or shoulder. Even when they know that only "tincture of time" will soothe your aching joints, doctors will often give you a cortisone shot. They do this even though research suggests very strongly that cortisone does not significantly improve healing for any of these painful conditions and may even speed joint deterioration.

So before you visit a doctor for help with a painful joint or spine, do a bit of research online to find out if the pain you are dealing with is one where a cortisone shot could be effective. If it isn't, don't let anyone talk you into letting them give you one.

If you have a condition where you will have to take corticosteroids for a long time, ask your doctor to refer you to an endocrinologist who can prescribe you the insulin you will need to keep your blood sugars from spending all their time at the extremely elevated levels that will damage your body. By this I mean readings of 250 mg/dl {13.9} or higher that won't come down no matter what you do. I have heard from people eating ketogenic diets who were still seeing very high blood sugars while on long-term corticosteroid therapy. Those very high blood sugars wouldn't come down with anything but a lot of insulin.

If your blood sugars remain elevated even after you have stopped taking a corticosteroid drug, try taking a small dose of Co-enzyme Q10 for a week and see if this helps lower them. That supplement may reverse some changes the cortisone drugs make to your mitochondria.

Will Hormone Replacement Improve or Worsen My Blood Sugar?

Hormone replacement may either raise or lower blood sugar, depending on which particular hormones you take and how your individual metabolism responds to them. So it isn't possible to make any categorical statements about them.

The specific hormones you take make a big difference. I was once prescribed a compounded mix of "bioidentical" hormones that pushed my post-meal blood sugar up a shocking 100 mg/dl {5.6} after I took a single pill. Another formulation I took for many years seemed to lower my blood sugar. Now my insurance is making me take yet another preparation that is doing a great job counteracting unpleasant meno-pausal symptoms but is also seems to be pushing my blood sugar up slightly, especially when I'm fasting.

For me, it's worth putting up with this, because estrogen replacement makes a huge difference not only in my health but in how well my brain works. Without it, my memory becomes a real problem, which is a serious concern now that I've reached the deceptively named "golden years." Other women may not see enough of a benefit when they take replacement hormones to make the hit on their blood sugars worth it.

Men with Type 2 Diabetes need to be very careful about supplementing with testosterone, as that kind of supplementation has been associated with a higher risk of heart attack. The problems that lead men to supplement with "T" are often caused by diabetic nerve damage and can be reversed by cutting back on carbohydrates for a year or so.

My Diabetes Is Getting Worse Despite Diet, Drugs, and Insulin What Should I Do?

As explained earlier, if you have had diabetes for less than five years, it's possible you have a slow developing form of autoimmune diabetes, LADA, that requires that you be treated for Type 1 rather than Type 2. Doctors can often misdiagnose middle aged people who are carrying a bit of weight with Type 2 when they really have this slow form of Type 1. This slow onset form older people get usually takes up to five years to get to the point where the person who has it is completely insulin dependent. This is very different from the form of autoimmune diabetes children and teens get, which can proceed to total insulin dependency after a period of only a few weeks.

There are simple tests that any endocrinologist can order and interpret that will make it clear if you are having the kind of autoimmune attack that will lead to full insulin dependency. As devastating as it may be to be given that diagnosis, it will allow you to qualify for better diabetes care. People with Type 1 Diabetes are prescribed much more effective insulin regimens, as well as devices like insulin pumps and continual glucose monitors that can help you maintain excellent control. Most insurers won't provide people with Type 2 Diabetes any of these devices. People with Type 1 also qualify for the kind of robust diabetes education from a highly trained Certified Diabetes Educator that teach you how to use insulin properly so you can maintain very tight control.

If you are diagnosed with autoimmune diabetes, you may also be able to benefit in the future from the beta cell regeneration and transplantation techniques that are advancing dramatically, or from an artificial pancreas. People with Type 2 will never have access to these extremely effective procedures or tools because there are too many of us.

If you've had Type 2 Diabetes for longer than five years, it is unlikely you have the autoimmune form of diabetes. Only a skilled endocrinologist will be able to figure out what, exactly, is causing your blood sugar control to be so difficult. Make an appointment to see one at whatever is the hospital associated with the best medical school in your region.

Chapter Nine

How Can I Heal My Complications?

I Had a Really High Blood Sugar Am I Doomed?

I often hear from people who are panicking because they've gone through a couple days when they've let their blood sugar rise way above the levels that can cause complications and now are afraid that they've inflicted serious damage on themselves.

They haven't. It takes a long time for high blood sugars to destroy your organs: decades, not weeks. Small lapses should not leave permanent scars.

So relax. No one with diabetes can hit their blood sugar targets all the time — at least none of us who isn't also diagnosed with obsessive compulsive disorder. You don't have to be perfect. You just have to hit that healthy blood sugar target more often then not.

A few highs each week won't doom you, though few highs *each day* are a different matter. Those do lead to complications over time, even those in the high prediabetic levels. So you don't want to get too relaxed. It's all too easy to let an occasional high now and then morph into a daily high that turns into a high after every meal.

But the great mercy of diabetes is how slowly it wreaks its havoc. If you've lost control, just get back on the wagon. You can still make dramatic improvements in your health years after your diagnosis.

Can I Reverse All the Damage from Diabetes with Tight Control?

Much of the damage caused by years of exposure to high blood sugars is reversible, but sadly not all. Dead nerves grow back at the rate of one millimeter a day, so over the course of a year or two you can undo a lot of the nerve damage caused by diabetes. This means you can cure painful feet, sexual dysfunction due to nerve damage, and, over a very long time, damage to the autonomic nerves that control heart beat.

Early kidney damage appears to be reversible, too, up to a certain point. I have heard from people who have recovered kidney function even after being diagnosed with serious kidney damage, though there does come a point where the damage has gone too far. Even the best blood sugar control can't reverse end stage kidney disease. It can, however, make a transplanted kidney last a lot longer.

Early changes to the retina can be improved, though there may be a temporary worsening before that improvement occurs. However, research shows that even people who experience that worsening in their retinas after they get better control still end up with their eyes in far better shape a decade later than do those who don't make that effort.

The complications that seem to be the most resistant to reversing are those that harden tissues that don't regenerate and make them become "crispy." The larger blood vessels, tendons, and vertebral discs seem to be areas where damage from previous exposure to high blood sugar may not be reversible.

That's why if your arteries have already stiffened up and are lined with plaque you may not be able to undo all the damage and will have to continue to do what your cardiologist tells you to do—except for the part about how you should be avoiding natural saturated fats and eating all those healthy whole grains and bananas!

Do All People with Diabetes Have to Get Heart Disease?

Doctors will tell you that people with diabetes always develop heart disease, but if you've read this far, I'm sure you've figured out that this is because the mediocre blood sugar control most doctors promote makes heart disease inevitable. The good news is that there is nothing about a diabetes diagnosis that dooms you to developing heart disease. Like the classic diabetic complications, heart disease is linked extremely tightly to how high your blood sugar rises. Keep your blood sugar in the near normal range and you can preserve your cardiovascular health, too.

What is really interesting about heart disease is that lots of people get it who never are given a diabetes diagnosis. But as was mentioned when we discussed the A1C earlier, research has shown that the link between blood sugar levels and heart disease isn't confined to people with diabetes. When huge, supposedly normal populations were studied, the researchers found that as the average A1C rose in these people, their risk of having a heart attack rose, too. People whose A1Cs neared 6% had about twice the risk of those whose A1Cs were below 5%, but as long as their A1Cs remained in the 5% range their risk was still fairly small. It only began to become significant as it went over 6%. At the 7.0% A1C most doctors consider to be "good enough for someone with diabetes" the risk is four times what it would be at 4.6%.

A1C might be predictive because some research suggests that glucose bonds to LDL molecules in our bloodstream just as it does to our hemoglobin. This appears to make the LDL stickier and more likely to cause trouble.

Other research has found that the changes in our arteries that lead to hardening appear to begin when people's blood sugars one hour after the start of a glucose tolerance test rise over 155 mg/dl {8.6}. That is a number that the ADA diagnostic criteria define as completely normal. But given how closely heart attack risk tracks that A1C, you have to wonder how normal they really are.

Obviously, there are quite a few other factors that can lead to a person developing heart disease that have nothing to do with blood sugar. Smoking is one, so are lots of different genes we may have inherited. But the data certainly suggests that if you can keep your blood sugars under 155 mg/dl one hour after eating, much of the time, you are a lot less likely to develop heart disease. You may even end up less likely to have a heart attack than your "normal" neighbor.

Unfortunately, most of us don't get a diabetes diagnosis—or even a diagnosis of prediabetes—until our blood sugars have been rising much higher than this for many years, so we may indeed already have stiffening in our arteries, plaque, and inflammation. But most people with diabetes, even those with the mediocre control doctors recommend, do not keel over with heart attacks until they are well past middle age. Metformin appears to prevent heart attacks, too, which is why it should be prescribed before any other diabetes drug.

The fact that diabetes is being diagnosed a bit earlier in the 2010s than it was twenty years ago and that more patients are taking metformin may explain why a study conducted in the early 2010s, which had been designed to study heart attacks in people with diabetes, was unable to achieve statistically significant results because not enough of the people with diabetes in the study had had heart attacks. This was very encouraging news for all of us.

What Tests Can Tell Me If I Am at Higher Risk Than Normal People for a Heart Attack?

Most doctors use the cholesterol test alone to assess your risk of heart attack. But half the people who have heart attacks have normal cholesterol test results. Others, like my dad, whose cholesterol was measured at 340 mg/dl {8.8} when he was in his 70s, live to be 100. My dad did have a heart attack at age 98, but he survived it. So it looks like cholesterol test results do a poor job of predicting heart attacks.

The triglyceride fraction reported by some cholesterol tests appears a bit more predictive. Triglyceride is just a fancy word for fat. In this case it refers to the fat which floats around in your blood until it is burned for energy, stored in fat cells, or deposited in your arteries. Having a lot of triglyceride in your blood does seem to be a warning sign that you are heading in an unhealthy direction. Keep in mind that it appears to be the carbs you eat, not the fats, that turn into triglycerides during digestion. People eating very low carbohydrate diets usually eat a lot of fat but still have very low triglyceride levels.

Another useful test that may give some insight into how likely you are to have a heart attack is the cardiac specific CRP test (cs-CRP). This test provides a measure of the inflammation in your arteries. High cs-CRP suggests high inflammation. People who have this kind of inflammation in their arteries probably should take a statin drug, as it appears that what statins do is lower this kind of inflammation.

Yet another test that might be helpful if you need to assess your risk of a heart attack is the coronary calcium scan. A study of veterans with Type 2 Diabetes found that those whose coronary calcium scores were under 100 were able to dramatically lower the risk of having a heart attack over the next seven years by aggressively lowering their blood sugar. With higher scores the results were less impressive.

And don't forget the A1C test. Though as we explained earlier, it may not always accurately estimate your actual blood sugar levels over the previous three months, when it comes close, it gives a pretty good measure of your heart disease risk unless you are one of those people whose A1C is always much lower than their post-meal blood sugars would predict it should be. A person with an A1C of 7.0% has four times the risk of having a heart attack as someone with one of 5.0%.

Incidentally, it was this finding that motivated a group of us who used to participate in the alt.support.diabetes newsgroup to aim for A1Cs in the 5% range and call ourselves "The 5% Club."

Why Do I Keep Getting a Stabbing Pain on My Left Side?

If you don't know why you are having a pain that could be a heart attack, don't guess or consult Dr. Google. If a pain lasts more than a few minutes or gets much worse, call the ambulance. Otherwise, make an appointment so your doctor can make sure it isn't being caused by something going on in your heart. Your family doctor will usually give you an EKG in the office to check this out.

If you get a clean bill of heart health and you are taking metformin, you might be experiencing a known side effect of metformin caused by the way it irritates the stomach lining. But quite a few people who are having actual heart attacks dismiss them as heartburn. So don't draw any conclusions about repeated episodes of mild pain in the left side of your chest until your doctor has checked out your heart.

Why Does Diabetes Damage Nerves?

Your nerves are made up of cells called neurons. These cells, like most other living cells, are dependent on tiny blood vessels called capillaries for the oxygen and glucose that they need in order to function. When your blood sugar is high for long periods of time, two things happen that limit the ability of these capillaries to bring oxygen and glucose to the nerves.

The first is that high blood sugars clog the tiny vessels. At damagingly high blood sugars, that extra sugar makes blood thicker, which makes it harder for it to flow through capillaries. Long term exposure to high blood sugar over time also damages the walls of the capillaries, making them stiffen up and become more prone to the formation of plaques. The stiff capillary walls eventually become fragile and are more likely to rupture. Though the tiny bleeds this causes may not seem all that important — unless they are happening in your brain in which case they cause mini-strokes — they eventually destroy the capillary.

Without the oxygen and glucose supply these capillaries were delivering, the nerves start dying too. The smallest ones die first, and then over time the larger ones, with larger blood supplies, start failing too.

Lowering your blood sugar to normal levels will restore the normal flow of blood to capillaries if you are in the earlier stages of diabetic nerve damage. This will, in turn allow nerves to heal that are fed by those capillaries. Structural damage to the capillaries will take longer to be repaired, but they do improve. Since the nerves of the autonomic nervous system that controls things like digestion and blood pressure are larger and fed by larger blood vessels, they may take longer to heal up, though some reports suggest that if you keep your blood sugar normal for a few years they, too, will heal.

Why Have My Feet Stopped Hurting Though My Blood Sugar Is Still Really High?

When your feet first start hurting it's because high blood sugars are damaging your nerves. But after a certain point the nerves start to die. Numbness then replaces pain, and you may feel better, but you're actually getting worse. That's because your nerves are what tell the rest of your immune system that something is wrong so that your immune system can send in specialized cells to fight off any invading organisms and rebuild damaged tissues.

Numb nerves no longer notice the tiny cuts that usually heal without any attention, allowing them to become portals for invading bacteria. Eventually you end up with the dreadful, deep and gaping, impossible-to heal-wounds that lead to diabetic amputations.

If your nerves are numb you will have to examine your feet daily or have a helper do that for you to check for even the tiniest scratch. These must be carefully treated with antibacterial ointment and bandaged. Call your doctor if any cut doesn't show signs of healing within a week.

And stop making excuses for ignoring your blood sugar. Numb feet are the last warning you get before irreversible organ damage begins to occur!

What Should I Do About the Terrible Pain in My Feet?

The only safe way to heal painful feet caused by diabetic nerve damage is to lower your blood sugar to normal levels.

This works. I have heard from plenty of people over the years who have pulled it off. But doctors won't tell you this because they rarely, if ever, see people who are able to cure their nerve pain in this way. The pills they prescribe aren't able to drop blood sugar levels low enough to get their patients' blood sugar down to the range where nerves will begin to heal as long as patients are still eating those high carbohydrate diets.

So since doctors don't see patients with diabetes who achieve normal blood sugars, they assume the damage is permanent and simply prescribe pills that they believe will help patients cope with the pain.

To achieve the normal blood sugar levels that will heal your nerves you will probably have to cut your carbohydrates way, way down — lower than the intake level people can use to prevent this complication from occurring. If you can keep your blood sugar spikes under 120 mg/dl {6.7}, your nerves should begin to heal if your nerve damage was, indeed, caused by diabetic nerve damage.

A ketogenic diet may be the best approach for doing this, as it will lower your blood sugar better than other diets. Some people will also need to take metformin to help reduce insulin resistance so they can reach totally normal blood sugar levels. Others may need a basal insulin.

Some people have reported that even after their nerves stopped hurting, their pain returns if they let their blood sugars spike over 140 mg/dl {7.8} for any significant period of time.

How Long Does It Take to Heal Damaged Nerves?

This depends on how badly they have been damaged. If you have had diabetes for a long time both tiny nerve fibers that branch off the larger nerve trunks and the thicker trunks may have been damaged, which will take a lot longer to heal—though if you are patient they will.

Reports from people who have cleared up painful feet by lowering their blood sugars suggest that you should start seeing results at about three months, though if you have had nerve pain for a long time before you start working on better control it may take a year for all the pain to go away.

I have never seen any data as to how long it takes for damage to the larger nerves to heal.

This Pill Makes My Feet Stop Hurting Are They Getting Better?

Unfortunately, the pills doctors prescribe for the pain caused by diabetic nerve damage merely dull the pain without doing anything to heal the nerves. Over time the nerves will go numb, making you feel less pain but leaving you open to the terrible incurable infections that lead to amputation.

There is also evidence that because these drugs work on the brain in ways that are not well understood, it can be extremely hard to stop taking them. For all practical purposes they are addictive—though the drug companies have lobbied hard to keep doctors from using this term to describe them.

But many users report that they experience terrible withdrawal symptoms when they try to quite them—effects that are as bad as or worse than the nerve pain they originally took them for. One person I spoke with, who had suffered greatly during a prolonged Neurontin withdrawal, told me his doctor told him it would take a year until his intense, life-altering, withdrawal symptoms abated. They included sharp shooting pains that felt like electric shocks.

To treat your nerve pain while waiting for your nerves to heal, try over-the-counter Tylenol (a.k.a. acetaminophen or paracetamol). It is often very helpful for controlling nerve pains of all kinds and helps with pain from vertebral disc disease, too. It may be just as effective against diabetic nerve pain with far fewer side effects than the prescription drugs. Just don't drink alcohol while taking it, since the combination of this drug and alcohol can destroy your liver even at relatively modest alcohol intake levels. If you find this drug works, take the very lowest dose that gives you relief. The non-extra strength dose may even be enough.

Medical marijuana does not cause withdrawal symptoms, either. If it is legal where you live, it might be worth testing out a strain that is recommended for pain relief to see if it helps. Just be sure that it is not a strain that is also used to restore appetite or counteract nausea, as those strains will make you overeat.

Whatever you do, avoid the temptation to use opiates. The threat of addiction is just too high. They have their place when you take them briefly while recovering from surgery, but you are going to be living with diabetic nerve pain for long enough that using opiates is too likely to lead to abuse.

Whatever you find that helps with your nerve pain, don't settle for pain relief. Get to work healing up your nerves the way we just described in the previous answer.

I've Kept My Blood Sugar Down Why Do My Feet Still Hurt?

If lowering your blood sugar doesn't heal your foot pain, it may have been caused by damaged vertebral discs in your lower back. People with Type 2 Diabetes often suffer from bulging or ruptured discs. Usually, nerve pain caused by disc injuries shows up in only one leg or the other, not both at the same time. Diabetic nerve damage, in contrast, usually affects both feet simultaneously. But severe disc damage can sometimes affect both feet. It also causes numbness and tingling. So when a doctor knows you have a diabetes diagnosis, they may misdiagnose it as diabetic nerve pain.

I've contended with vertebral disc disease for decades and my advice is that if your foot pain is caused by your discs, resist the temptation to cure it with surgery unless it is intolerable. Studies have shown that people who wait out chronic disc pain end up in as good shape as those who have surgery. Within my own circle of acquaintances, those of us who have *not* had vertebral disc back surgery seem to be in much better shape twenty years later than those who did. I have been told that outcomes are better with neck surgeries for ruptured discs than back surgeries, but those I know who have had neck surgery still report that they have pain. The only time surgery is not negotiable is when there is visual evidence on an MRI that your spinal cord is being compressed.

There are other conditions that also cause nerves to deteriorate. Some are difficult or even impossible to diagnose. I get a certain amount of email from people with painful nerves who have completely normal blood sugars but are desperately hoping they have diabetes because neurologists have not been able to come up with any explanation for their nerve pain.

My Hands Tingle a Lot Is This from Diabetes?

As just mentioned, I often get mail from people who have a long list of symptoms they desperately hope have been caused undiagnosed diabetes. This is because their doctors have been unable to come up with any diagnosis that would explain what is causing their symptoms.

Most of them have completely normal blood sugars, but a surprising number of them have tingling in their arms they are sure is diabetic neuropathy though their feet are fine.

Tingling in your arms is very unlikely to be caused by diabetes unless you have been diagnosed with diabetes for long enough that both your feet are affected. Diabetic nerve damage almost always starts showing up first in your feet because the nerves that extend from your spine to your feet are the longest in the body. It is very unusual for diabetic neuropathy to show up first in the hands.

The neuropathy caused by uncontrolled diabetes is most likely to start out with pain and then numbness in the feet and sexual dysfunction. Over time these are followed by a slowdown in digestion, all of which happen before diabetes hand pain ever shows up.

Tingling in your hands but not your arms, or sudden numbness in your hands is often a sign of hyperventilation—extremely shallow fast breathing, which is something people do when they are very anxious.

Nerve pains down the arms that reach into the hands are much more likely to be caused by pinched nerves in the neck or bulging or ruptured vertebral discs in the neck.

Vitamin B12 deficiency is one last thing that can cause weird nerve pains throughout your body. Eating vegan or vegetarian diets can lead to the development of this deficiency. The nerve symptoms it causes are not reversible—another very good reason to be very cautious about believing the hype about how vegan diets are good for people with diabetes.

If you have been taking metformin for more than four years, your doctor should test your B12 levels and repeat that test every couple years in the future to rule B12 deficiency, as metformin may inhibit your ability to absorb Vitamin B12 from food.

My doctor says that sublingual high dose Vitamin B12 pills can restore Vitamin B12 levels. Other sources say that shots may be needed.

What Causes Diabetic Amputations?

Diabetic amputations happen after people develop infected wounds on their feet that won't heal. These wounds turn into diabetic ulcers — terrible rotted out holes in your flesh that may extend down to the bone and, eventually, turn gangrenous.

This usually happens to people whose blood sugar has been extremely high for years — think A1Cs of 10% and higher — often much higher. These blood sugar levels originally cause nerve pain, but after a while the nerves become so damaged that they stop transmitting pain and go numb. This is a relief to the person who has been feeling that horrid nerve pain, but the loss of the feedback from those nerves has terrible consequences.

Not only do you no longer notice when you've cut yourself, often quite severely, but your immune system relies on your nerves to inform it that something is going on so it can send immune system cells to fight off any invaders. Cut your foot when it has normal nerves in it, and the pain you feel sends a message to your brain that will prompt a response that results in your immune system swiftly sending out cells to defend you against any bacteria that came in with whatever caused you pain. You can tell this happened because you experience inflammation at the site of a cut as the immune system does its work.

But with dead nerves, the immune system may not notice an invader until the damage is severe enough that other larger nerves, higher up report it. Furthermore, by the time your nerves are damaged enough to have become numb, something else, equally troublesome has happened: the blood supply to those nerves and the tissues surrounding them has become scanty because your blood vessels have become clogged, stiff, and possibly full of plaque that causes them to close up. Since you need intact blood vessels to bring infection-fighting immune cells to those tissues, even if the brain gets the signal that something is wrong, the healing cells may never be able to get to the infected tissue.

None of this is likely to become a problem for anyone recently diagnosed with diabetes who keeps their blood sugar at reasonably safe levels. If you already have some neuropathy in your feet, congratulate yourself when it is painful rather than numb. If you have numbness, don't panic, either. Work on healing those nerves. You can do it. Typically the people who develop infections bad enough to lead to amputation have experienced decades of exposure to very high blood sugars day in and day out before their infections have gone out of control.

But this should make it clear why, if you have numbness in your feet, it is extremely important to protect them from little cuts of any type that could become infected, whether they are caused by athletes' foot or a stubbed toe. Don't wear shoes that rub anywhere against your feet. Wear sandals at the beach. Put antibiotic ointment on any break in the skin no matter how tiny. Have someone examine your feet every few days to make sure there isn't something you missed.

Smoking also damages the same blood vessels that are under siege from diabetes, so if you have nerve damage in your feet it is essential that you stop smoking, as the double whammy of uncontrolled diabetes and smoking is much more likely to lead to severe infections that could lead to amputation.

If you do get any kind of ulcer on your feet, demand very aggressive treatment from your doctor. Ideally you should see a wound care specialist rather than be treated by your family doctor. Wound care doctors have much more expertise in treating infected wounds that won't heal than do general practitioners. The earlier any small ulcer is seen by a wound specialist, the more likely you are to avoid amputation. If your family doctor brushes off your concerns, find a new one.

Why Do My Feet Hurt Worse Now That I've Lowered My Blood Sugar?

When your nerves are badly damaged they go numb, which gives you a strange feeling from time to time, like something is stuck between your toes, but mostly goes unnoticed. However, when you lower your blood sugar to healthy levels for a few months and those nerves begin to heal, they start working again. When they do they often hurt like the dickens or itch, depending on where the nerve is.

This will pass as the nerve gets healthier. So when you feel that kind of pain after a long period of nerve numbness take it as a good sign. Your feet are getting healthier.

Why Does My Heating Pad Warn Not to Use It If I'm Diabetic?

If diabetes has killed off enough nerves, you may not be able to sense when a heating pad has become hot enough to burn your skin. Hence the warning. It is mostly put on labels to protect the heating pad company from lawsuits.

If you don't have severe diabetic nerve damage, this shouldn't be an issue for you.

Why Does the Sign at the Gym Tell Me to Stay out of the Hot Tub?

People who have followed mainstream medical advice almost always have nerve damage in the vagus nerve, which is a long nerve that controls several functions you can't control consciously, like your digestion, your heart rate, and the response of the immune system. It is part of what is called the autonomic nervous system. When your vagus nerve is not working correctly, you are much more likely to faint, hence people with diabetes who have damaged vagus nerves are more likely than others to pass out and drown in a hot tub.

If you don't have episodes of dizziness and fainting, your blood sugars are normal, and your nerves are fine, this isn't a concern. But if you have serious problems with diabetic nerve pain, it is possible that your vagus nerve is affected, too. In that case, don't ever go into a hot tub alone.

In the good old days hot tubs were really hot, which was wonderful for those of us with sore muscles. But that heat posed another threat to people with diabetes, because numb nerves in their feet could make them unaware that water was hot enough to burn their tissues. Owners of public hot tubs are now so afraid of being sued that the water temperature in most of them is low enough that taking chill is a more likely outcome than burned feet.

Is Diabetes Causing My Digestive Symptoms?

The vagus nerve we just mentioned is a long nerve that stretches from your brain all the way down to your colon. One of its functions is to control the valve in your stomach that lets food move from the stomach into the duodenum. Like any nerve, the vagus nerve can be damaged by long exposure to diabetic high blood sugars.

This particular form of diabetic nerve damage usually takes decades to develop, but when it does what happens is that the valve at the bottom of your stomach starts behaving unpredictably and food may sit for far longer than usual in your stomach without digesting. This will make you feel unpleasantly full. It may even make you feel nauseated. Because your food isn't digesting it may take an extra hour or two until you experience the blood sugar spike that occurs after meals. When those spikes do appear, they may occur very unpredictably. If this is the case, it will be impossible to use fast-acting insulin or a pill that causes your pancreas to secrete insulin without a much greater risk of having a hypo.

The medical term for this kind of stomach problem is gastroparesis — paralyzed stomach. There are several other conditions unrelated to diabetes that can also cause this gastroparesis. They have nothing to do with damage from high blood sugars. I have known someone who developed it after a virus. In that case it healed up over a decade.

Some drugs and supplements also can slow down digestion or bring it to a near halt. Too much magnesium can have this effect. So can taking Pepcid for heartburn. If you notice that you are nauseated a lot while taking a supplement or over the counter heartburn pill, cut back on the dose and see if the problem goes away.

While your stomach is emptying slowly, don't take insulin or drugs that cause you to secrete insulin, because the combination of gastroparesis and insulin can cause very nasty hypos when the insulin hits your blood before a meal's worth of glucose does.

Why Does Everyone I Know with Diabetes Have Heartburn?

There is no one answer here, as several factors might explain the problem. Here they are, in no particular order:

Middle aged people often develop a condition called hiatal hernia where the upper part of the stomach has bulged up through the hole in the diaphragm. Doctors may tell you this happens because you are overweight, but it happened to me when I was at a totally normal weight and BMI. Pregnancy can also cause this. So can coughing. Once it happens, stomach acid may irritate esophageal tissues, especially when you lie down, because the valve that usually keeps acid in the stomach doesn't work properly any more.

A sensitivity to wheat gluten is another reason many people develop heartburn. While this isn't classic gluten intolerance, it's one reason it might be a good idea to try a gluten free or wheat free diet for a few weeks to see if it cures persistent heartburn. My experience has been that after a couple of years going almost completely wheat-free the problem went away and for many years afterwards I could eat wheat again without heartburn. Eventually, it came back.

Another reason for persistent heartburn, unfortunately, may be metformin, which can irritate the stomach lining. Try taking a few weeks off metformin to see if that eliminates your heartburn. If it does, try taking your metformin only on a full stomach. If that doesn't help, a low dose of Pepcid might be useful, but be aware that it is on the list of drugs that might raise the risk of dementia in older people. Prilosec has very troubling side effects and can be very tough to get off of, so it is a poorer choice if you are battling relentless heartburn.

There is one last reason why some people with diabetes may get heartburn that doesn't respond well to medication. People with diabetes are more prone to fungal infections like vaginal yeast and athlete's foot. It turns out that the same organisms that cause vaginal yeast are capable of infecting your esophagus. This kind of heartburn, unlike the usual kind, does not clear up when you cut out wheat. I have had one of these infections, diagnosed via gastroscopy. The main thing that was different about that yeast infection was that when I stopped metformin, cut way down on carbs and ate more fat, it got worse, not better. Run of the mill heartburn usually goes away if you eat a ketogenic diet.

The faddy "yeast free" diet that eliminates all fermented foods will not cure this. That diet appears to cure heartburn only because most people who eat it stop eating bread and wheat gluten is a common cause of heartburn. But the yeasts used to ferment beer or raise dough are completely different species. They are more different from candida than you are from your pet cat. You can't make a candida infection go away by eating lots of yogurt, either. These candida organisms burrow down deep into your esophageal or gastric tissues. It takes massive doses of ketoconazole to kill them off, once you are diagnosed with this kind of infection. Then you will have to take heartburn pills for at least three months to let the damaged tissues heal.

People with normal blood sugars who swallow these kinds of fungi don't seem to get infected by them, so it is likely that if you normalize your blood sugar you will have less trouble with this kind of infection in the future.

Is Athlete's Foot a Diabetic Complication?

When your blood sugar is high, the damp, airless creases anywhere on your body become more attractive to fungal invaders, as all your secretions, including your sweat, have extra glucose in them that nourishes them. So recurrent bouts of hard-to-treat athletes' foot can be a warning sign that a person's blood sugars are higher than they should be. Lowering those blood sugars to normal levels should make it easier to permanently eradicate the problem.

If you have diabetic nerve pain or numbness in your feet, be aggressive in treating any hint of athletes foot with antifungal cream applied daily. If you don't see improvement, ask your doctor for one of the stronger prescription drugs. The cracks in your skin these fungal infections cause can lead to slow-healing infections.

Are Vaginal Yeast Infections Another Complication?

Vaginal yeast infections go virtually unmentioned in every discussion of diabetes I've ever read, but for countless women they are an early sign that blood sugars have gone out of control. Lowering your blood sugar to normal limits may make it easier to control yeast, but if you have already been colonized by hardy strains, it may take a lot of work to get rid of them permanently. Several days worth of ketoconazole, which only a doctor can prescribe, can often get the job done.

If that doesn't work, give capsules of boric acid you insert into your vagina a try. You'll find directions on how to do this on this WebMD page: **http://www.webmd.com/women/tc/boric-acid-for-vaginal-yeast-infection-topic-overview.** You don't need to order the very expensive bottles of boric acid sold by supplement companies. Plain Humco boric acid, which you can buy in bottles at some pharmacies and from Amazon, will work just fine. If you have trouble getting the capsules to melt, use one of the plastic inserters that come with yeast cream or estrogen cream to insert the boric acid.

Are My Recurrent Urinary Tract Infections a Diabetes Complication?

Urinary tract infections are a known side effect of the new SGLT-2 inhibitor drugs like Invokana, Jardiance, and Farxiga. Otherwise, recurrent urinary tract infections aren't considered a classic diabetic complication, as plenty of women with normal blood sugars get these, too. They usually result from bacteria working their way into the bladder where they form tough biofilms that make them resistant to antibiotics. However, if you have high blood sugar, these bacteria get more food to spur their growth, which can make infections worse, as is true of any other bacterial infection. It is possible that, like recurrent vaginal infections, recurrent urinary tract infections might be a very early signal that your blood sugar after meals is higher than normal.

If you get these, don't treat them with sugary cranberry juice. Cranberry juice is yet another debunked cure that is worthless and you don't need the sugar. Antibiotics are usually needed, but they have to be the right ones. Since some persistent urinary tract infections are actually urethral infections, if the usual drugs prescribed for urinary tract infections don't help, you will need to take one of the few antibiotics, like doxycycline, that are able to reach the urethra. Most drugs that heal bladder infections are useless for urethral urinary tract infections. Many family doctors are not aware of this.

If you start getting urethral infections and are at an age where menopause is an issue, estrogen cream may build up the tissues in a way that prevents them from being so prone to infection.

Is Erectile Dysfunction a Diabetic Complication?

There is an old saying among doctors that "The penis is the divining rod of the cardiovascular system." When it is working well, chances are good that so are the rest of your arteries. Conversely, if it starts to fail it's a flashing red light signaling that all is not well with the rest of your blood vessels.

Sexual response requires unimpeded blood flow and healthy nerves, both of which erode after years of exposure to elevated blood sugars, including those that only rise into the high prediabetic range.

If doctors better understood the connection between heart disease and blood sugar they would prescribe blood sugar meters rather than Viagra when male patients came in complaining of erectile dysfunction. That's because, as is the case with so many of the remedies doctors prescribe, Viagra just masks the underlying condition. It doesn't heal it.

If you have diabetes or prediabetes and treat your erectile dysfunction only by taking Viagra, over time your nerves and small blood vessels will continue to deteriorate to where Viagra will no longer work. And of course, the rest of your nerves and blood vessels will keep deteriorating, too.

Lowering high blood sugars, as you have read over and over again in these pages, will heal nerve damage. As a woman, I have no personal experience with this particular dividing rod, so I have to take the word of others about whether lowering blood sugars can improve male sexual performance. Dr. Bernstein says that erectile dysfunction can be reversed if it is mainly caused by nerve damage but that if it is caused by damage to larger blood vessels reversal may be tougher.

Women's sexual response is just as dependent on healthy nerves and blood vessels as is men's. It's just not as evident when the system has started to fail. If you are in your forties or older, doctors usually blame any sexual problems you experience on menopause—as they do just about anything else that is wrong with you. And it is true that if you are not taking hormone replacement therapy, your sexual response may decline even without blood sugar-related problems. But it's likely that getting better control over your blood sugars will heal any damage caused by failing nerves.

Unfortunately, the diabetes drug metformin can sometimes, though by no means always, cause estradiol (estrogen) and testosterone levels to drop in people of either sex. This might be something you have to live with if metformin makes it easier to maintain much more normal blood sugars. I have not received any reports that metformin completely shut down anyone's sexual response. So this isn't a reason to stop taking the drug.

Why Does Diabetes Damage Kidneys?

High blood sugars appear to damage the tiny blood vessels in the kidney that filter out many of the chemicals in your blood that don't belong there. At a certain point, so many of these are damaged that the kidney allows dangerous levels of chemicals to accumulate in your blood and you need to go on dialysis to remove them.

Research has found that it is not only exposure to high blood sugars that causes this damage. The kidneys are also very sensitive to large changes in the concentration of glucose in the blood. So for example, blood sugars that spike up to 350 mg/dl {19.4} and then drop down to 180 mg/dl {10} appear to be more damaging than blood sugars that sit at 250 mg/dl much of the day but don't fluctuate as much.

As is the case with all the other complications we've discussed, early kidney damage also appears to get underway when your blood sugars remain over 140 mg/dl {7.8} for more than a couple hours after a meal.

Kidney failure is also caused by high blood pressure, which also afflicts many people with diabetes. So to preserve your kidneys, you should do what you can to keep your blood pressure down, not just your blood sugar.

How Can I Tell If I Have Diabetic Kidney Disease?

One you have a diabetes diagnosis, your doctor should order a urine test that measures how much protein is leaking into your urine. This is called the microalbumin test. If the result comes back even slightly abnormal, assume you have early kidney disease and get serious about lowering your blood sugar. Early changes in the kidney are reversible.

Make sure you get a copy of the actual test result from your doctor. This will present your reading along with the lab's reference range. If your reading is at the top of the reference range or is flagged as "high," take it very seriously.

All too often, doctors will not bother to mention slightly abnormal lab results to you. Sometimes this is appropriate, because a single lab test can sometimes come in with a very slightly elevated reading, which goes back to normal the next time you are tested. But if a slightly abnormal result persists or becomes a bit more abnormal a few months later, something bad is likely to be happening.

Your doctor may also not mention a slightly abnormal result because doctors expect people with diabetes to develop all the classic diabetic complications and there isn't any drug they can prescribe that will reverse early diabetic kidney disease.

But since early kidney disease can, indeed, be reversed by achieving normal blood sugars, you should never ignore even a slightly abnormal microalbumin test, but should use it as motivation to work harder on regaining normal blood sugar control.

Can I Reverse Kidney Damage Caused by Diabetes?

Research has found that diabetic kidney damage begins to show up in groups of people when their A1Cs go over 6.0%, so to reverse diabetic kidney damage, it is obvious you would have to achieve much better control than the 7.0-7.5% most doctors think is all you need.

I have heard from people I've met online who have reversed kidney damage by adhering to strict low carb diets for several years. Dr. Richard K. Bernstein also claims in his books to have reversed his own, fairly advanced, kidney damage years ago, too. He's well into his 80s and still using the kidneys he was born with despite having been diagnosed with diabetes in 1946. So I trust his word on this.

Because blood sugar swings are as damaging as high blood sugars, to heal up your kidneys, you will have to not only lower your blood sugar but also keep the swings up and down as low as possible.

Your kidney function can also be damaged by taking too many over-the-counter painkillers, like Tylenol or ibuprofen. Some research has found that there seems to be a lifetime limit of how much of these drugs your kidneys can handle. So think twice about taking them, and if you really need one, take the very lowest dose that takes care of your pain. This often is a lot less than you might think.

There is one last issue that rarely gets mentioned even by people who obsess about every bite they put into their mouths. This is a shame, because it is essential information for anyone who is trying to keep their kidneys working. You need to avoid eating processed foods and drinks whose ingredients include inorganic phosphate additives. These ingredients include sodium phosphate, disodium phosphate, and calcium phosphate, but there are many others. As you learned on Page 117, the amount of these phosphate additives a person eats has been linked to their blood levels of these substances. High blood levels of phosphates are known to raise the risk of both kidney damage and heart disease.

They are discussed more fully on the web page Added Inorganic Phosphates Damage Your Kidneys and Cardiovascular System, which you'll find at **http://www.bloodsugar101.com/47759082.php**.

I Have Kidney Disease Does That Mean I Can't Eat a Low Carb Diet Because of the Protein?

Because there is so much protein in the urine of people with kidney disease it was long believed that it was the consumption of protein that caused kidney damage and that people with kidney damage should eat low protein diets. Eventually researchers proved that limiting protein did not prevent further damage to the kidney.

So it appears to be safe to eat normal amounts of protein when you have kidney disease. But keep the emphasis on "normal." A healthy low carb diet should not be a high protein diet. It should be an *adequate protein* diet with a normal amount of protein. The carbs you have removed should be replaced by healthy fats. Fat does not have a harmful effect on the kidneys where blood sugars are very well controlled.

There Are Foam Bubbles in My Urine Does This Mean I Have Kidney Damage?

Foam in the toilet bowl after you urinate is listed as one of the symptoms of kidney disease. But don't panic if you see a few bubbles. They may be caused by something else. If you have had a microalbumin test that came back fine, you should have nothing to worry about.

If you haven't had one of these tests recently, mention this symptom to your doctor the next time you see him and ask your doctor to run a microalbumin test to calm your worries.

What Causes Diabetic Blindness?

High blood sugars damage the tiny blood vessels that supply your retinas, which are the nerves that carry visual signals to your brain. When this happens, new blood vessels start growing at the site of the damage that are fragile, leaky, and abnormally dense. Doctors call this new growth proliferation. It is considered an early stage of diabetic retinopathy, which is what doctors call diabetic eye disease.

Damaged blood vessels in the eye can leak fluid into the macula, the center of the retina, which results in a condition called "macular edema." The drugs Avandia and Actos also turned out to promote the development of macular edema. Macular edema may cause blurry vision, but so can other more benign factors, like allergies affecting your corneas.

You can do a quick test at home to determine if there is a problem with your macula by looking at the Amsler Grid you will find on this website: **https://nei.nih.gov/health/macular-edema/fact_sheet**. If you see anything worrisome, make an appointment with an ophthalmologist to get it checked out.

After many years of exposure to high blood sugars, the fragile, abnormal blood vessels in the eye may rupture badly enough that blood leaks into the clear substance that fills your eyeball. This can be treated by focusing lasers on the bleeding vessels to seal them, but this treatment damages the retina, too.

If too much blood fills the eye surgeons can replace the jelly that fills it. But eventually, if blood sugars remain high, the damaged blood supply damages the retinas to the point where they stop working.

Fortunately, diabetic blindness has become much rarer among people with Type 2 Diabetes than it was in the 1990s, now that doctors don't routinely ignore very high A1Cs. However, many doctors still believe that it is impossible to completely prevent diabetic retinopathy from developing because their patients with the 7.0% A1Cs they recommend still develop some, though at a slower rate.

If you have early signs of retinopathy, take it very seriously, even if your doctor tells you that you aren't likely to go blind. The retina is the only place in your body where it is possible to see how well your blood vessels are doing without cutting you open. If the tiny blood vessels in your eyes are deteriorating, it's also likely that the ones in your brain aren't doing so well either. If the blood vessels in your brain are becoming fragile, your chances of having a stroke are rising, too.

So when you see your eye doctor, grill them about whether you have any signs of retinopathy, even the most trivial. Remember that most doctors expect people with diabetes to have early diabetic complications and may consider very mild retinopathy "good enough for someone with diabetes" and not even bother to mention it to you, though it will be entered into your medical records.

My Vision Keeps Getting Blurry Is Diabetes Making Me Blind?

Many of us will experience dramatic fluctuations in the sharpness of our vision when our blood sugar rises much higher or drops much lower then usual. This can be very frightening if you are worried about developing diabetic blindness.

But early retinopathy usually has no symptoms, so unless you've been told by a doctor that you have significant retinopathy, these sudden, disturbing changes in visual acuity are unlikely to be caused by retinal changes, and while they can be alarming, they don't pose a threat to your vision.

What causes these fluctuations is this: When your blood sugar goes high the concentration of glucose in the lens in your eye rises too, which alters the optical properties of that lens. When your blood sugar drops, your lens goes back to having its usual properties.

Whether or not you will notice these changes has a lot to do with how old you are and how flexible your lenses are. It generally becomes more of a problem when you are at the age where you need bifocals, since at that point your lenses have lost their elasticity.

High blood sugar is not the only factor that can make you wonder if you've put on someone else's glasses. Dry air can also affect the surface of the eye and change vision dramatically. So can dehydration. But because high blood sugars can make such a difference in your visual acuity, you may find yourself needing to get a new prescription after you have significantly lowered your blood sugar.

When you get your eyes examined for this new prescription, try to schedule your appointment for a time of day when your blood sugar is closest to the level it is at most of the time so that your prescription best matches your usual blood sugar.

WARNING: If you are taking insulin or one of the pills that stimulates insulin release (glipizide, glyburide, glibenclamide, repaglinide, etc.) and notice a sudden change in your vision, like a patch that has become wavy, a sudden appearance of sparkling lights, or a shrinking of your visual field, check your blood sugar immediately. These can be symptoms of a serious hypo—one where your blood sugar has dropped below 40 mg/dl {2.2}. If your blood sugar drops much lower you may pass out.

If this happens when you are driving, pull over immediately and check your blood sugar. If you are hypoing, take some of the glucose you should always keep in your car. Don't start driving again until you've determined that your blood sugar is over 85 mg/dl {4.7} and stable.

Why Did My Eyes Get Worse After I Lowered My Blood Sugar?

If your blood sugar has been very high for a very long time, some destructive chemicals will have built up within your eyes. Then when you lower your blood sugar, these chemicals leave your eyes, but they cause some further damage on the way out. This can cause some temporary worsening in your retinas.

There isn't any way to avoid this. Research has confirmed that it doesn't matter if you lower your blood sugar quickly or slowly. It still happens. Leaving your blood sugars high won't improve matters, as they will only make your retinopathy worse and lead to the build up of even more of these toxic chemicals.

However, even with some temporary worsening, years later you will end up with better vision than people who started out with the same degree of retinopathy as you did who did not lower their blood sugars. So don't let any temporary worsening worry you. The damage that is already done can't be completely undone, but you can stop any further damage from occurring.

How Do I Know If I Am Getting Diabetic Eye Disease?

The early damage diabetes does to your retinas has no symptoms. So the only way to know if you are have diabetic eye disease is to get a dilated eye examination from a professional. An optometrist can do a screening exam quite cheaply, but if they find any suggestion of diabetic eye disease they will tell you to see an ophthalmologist. Do so.

If the ophthalmologist sees a serious problem with your retina, they, in turn, will refer you to a retinologist, who is an even more highly-trained specialist. They are the only kind of doctor you should ever let perform any procedures on your retinas.

Is Dry Eye a Diabetic Complication?

Dry eye can be caused by a lot of things that have nothing to do with your blood sugar, like the hormonal changes of midlife, allergies, or low humidity in your home. But people with diabetes tend to have more problems with dry eye than others their age.

Several reasons have been suggested for this. One is that tears in people with diabetic blood sugars have more glucose in them, which may promote infection with micro-organisms that feed of this glucose. Another is that mild nerve damage may affect the system that controls eye-watering, so that not enough tears are secreted. The nerves at the surface of the eye, if damaged, may also become more sensitive.

Lowering your blood sugar to near normal levels should help dry eye if it is being caused by high blood sugars. Meanwhile, taking a small dose of fish oil or olive oil every day seems to help many people, as the extra oil seems to make its way into the tears that are secreted and helps them resist evaporation better.

Doctors will usually just suggest that you use artificial tears, but I have tried quite a few brands and have never found any of them to be of much use.

Are Cataracts a Diabetic Complication?

Cataracts are another of those conditions that are not considered classic diabetic complications, because plenty of people who haven't been diagnosed with diabetes get them too. But people with diabetes are more likely than others to get cataracts.

This is probably because the higher level of glucose in the lens—the same glucose that can make it harder to read when your blood sugar is high—promotes the crosslinking of proteins in the lens that causes them to cloud up.

Does Diabetes Cause Dementia?

Dementia is not one disease, but several, and the form of dementia most closely connected to diabetes is vascular dementia, where a person experiences numerous small strokes as tiny blood vessels in their brain rupture. These may be so small that they aren't even noticed, but over time they destroy brain tissue.

Where things get murkier is when we turn to other forms of dementia such as classic Alzheimer's, which is the dementia characterized by the presence of clumps of a protein called beta amyloid that form plaques throughout the brain. There seems to be an association between diabetes and classic Alzheimer's, but which causes which isn't clear. Recent research suggests that it may be the Alzheimer's disease that causes the deteriorating blood sugar control that is often found in people who have Alzheimer's, not the blood sugars causing the Alzheimer's. But so little is really understood about what causes Alzheimer's that you can safely ignore all the headlines. Honest scientists will tell you that we don't understand it well at all.

But the connection between vascular dementia and diabetic blood sugars is well understood, and since vascular dementia will make you just as demented as classic Alzheimer's, this is yet another thing that should motivate you to lower your blood sugars.

Though there is no research on what happens to people with diabetes who control their blood sugars into old age, I have run into several people who have lived to be very quite old with the severest form of diabetes—Type 1 diagnosed in childhood—whose brains have remained fully functional. Dr. Bernstein is the most famous example. He is still practicing medicine in his early 80s. Not so coincidentally, he has been maintaining normal blood sugars since the 1970s, when he became the first person with diabetes to ever own a blood sugar meter.

But he's not the only person with severe diabetes whose brain has lasted as long as needed. Several years ago I received an email from a man with Type 1 Diabetes who told me he was still going strong in his 90s. I asked him how he'd survived in so much better shape than his peers. In response, he explained that when he was diagnosed as a child, not long after the discovery of insulin, he was taught to eat as little carbohydrate as possible. This was how diabetes was always treated at the time. Later, when doctors started recommending that people with diabetes switch to eating low fat, high carbohydrate diets, he had been doing so well on his old diet that he kept on eating that way. So despite having had no access to a blood sugar meter for decades, he'd still been able to keep himself healthy.

Stories about one or two people don't prove anything. We all know pack a day smokers who lived to a great age, too. But for now, it's all we've got. It won't be until my generation of people with diabetes reach our nineties that there will be enough data about people who maintain very good control to draw any meaningful conclusions. Given how effective blood sugar control is for preventing the many other conditions caused by deteriorating blood vessels, it seems reasonable to hope that tight blood sugar control can allow more of us to die with all our marbles.

Why Do I Keep Getting Frozen Shoulders?

Frozen shoulder is caused by problems with the tendons that surround your shoulder. Frozen shoulders often occur as long as a decade before a person is officially diagnosed with diabetes and are definitely more common among people who are already diagnosed with diabetes. Frozen shoulders can be extremely painful, but unlike other diabetes-related conditions, they usually go away in a few months without any need for treatment.

Doctors often offer cortisone shots for a frozen shoulder, but the research suggests that they are not helpful except, perhaps, as a placebo. In fact, they may be harmful and actually weaken the tendons into which they have been injected. And of course, when you take a cortisone shot you risk having your blood sugar control worsen.

Doctors will also recommend physical therapy, but again, research shows that people who have this physical therapy—which can be quite painful and expensive—recover at the same rate as people who do nothing.

I have had two occurrences of frozen shoulder that healed up on their own in about three months. I also had one occurrence that did not heal up on its own, but remained very painful and difficult to move until I saw a very skilled acupuncturist who practices at our regional teaching hospital's pain clinic. After he gave me a second treatment, the shoulder suddenly unfroze, completely stopped hurting, and resumed working properly. The acupuncturist explained to me that sometimes muscles will go into spasm after a painful injury, even after the injury has healed and that when that is the case, acupuncture can make them relax. That said, acupuncture seems useful only after the initial inflammation has resolved. I have not found it useful when I tried it just a few weeks after developing a different frozen shoulder.

Are Other Tendon Problems a Diabetic Complication?

Tendons have very meager blood supplies even in healthy people, so when their tiny blood vessels become damaged by elevated blood sugars—even those in the prediabetic range—the damage shows up in them first.

Some other tendon problems that may occur in people with diabetes are carpal tunnel syndrome, tennis elbow, piriformis syndrome, and tarsal tunnel syndrome, which is the foot version of carpal tunnel syndrome.

If you get one of these you will have to wait it out. Do not try to "push through" a tendon injury. It requires rest to heal.

Several times I have one of these tendon issues flare up after I have lowered my blood sugar from a previous high, not while it was high. This makes me wonder if perhaps when blood sugars drop, some chemical change occurs in the tendon that is painful at first, though it then goes away.

The good news is that tendon problems do heal up if you give them time and don't overwork the joints involved.

Are My Mood Swings Caused by Diabetes?

Some people experience mood swings when their blood sugar is fluctuating strongly, though it is a stretch to say that diabetes causes mood swings. One interesting finding from research is that diabetes *does not* cause clinical depression.

For years doctors assumed there was a strong connection between the two because so many people with diabetes were also taking antidepressants. But the evidence showed, on closer analysis, that it seemed to be the antidepressants that were causing the diabetes, rather than the other way around.

The obvious conclusion from this is that people with blood sugar problems should not take antidepressants unless it is a matter of life and death, because they do appear to worsen blood sugar control, perhaps permanently. People with garden variety depression who do not take antidepressants turn out to get over it at the exact same rate as people who take them. Therapy with a skilled, empathic therapist can be even more helpful than drugs, too. It may cost more, but it won't mess up your metabolism.

Why Did My Doctor Say Diabetes Will Make My Surgery More Dangerous?

If your blood sugars have been running at the elevated levels that too many doctors think is "good enough for a diabetic" for several years, yes, you are more likely to have a post-operative infection and your surgical wounds may heal slowly. This is because of the damage that long years of exposure to high blood sugars can do to the small blood vessels that supply oxygen to healing tissues and carry the immune system cells that fight infection.

But you can improve your chances of a good recovery when you have surgery scheduled in the future by going on a strict low carb diet for as long as you can before that surgery and then sticking to that diet during the six weeks it takes to heal up after it. Eating more protein than usual after your surgery will also help your wounds heal faster, too.

Is Everything a Diabetic Complication?

Because diabetes can affect so many different organs and cause so many different symptoms, it's easy to start thinking that everything that could ever go wrong with you is caused by diabetes. But people with perfectly normal blood sugars do not live forever, and many of them, don't live as long as people with diabetes who keep their blood sugars under control.

There are quite a few pain syndromes, joint diseases, digestive disorders, brain syndromes, cancers, and inflammatory diseases that develop in people with perfectly normal blood sugars. Most people who have them can eat whatever they want, unlike people with diabetes. But that's because nothing they eat will make any improvement in their condition. They can't do a thing on their own to get rid of their symptoms or slow the rate at which they deteriorate. All they can do is take the drugs their doctors offer and hope that they work.

When I talk to people who have these kinds of diseases, I feel so lucky. How fine a thing it is that just by changing what I eat I can make such a huge difference in my health! The conclusion is inescapable: If you have to have a chronic condition, this is the one to have.

Not everyone is so fortunate!

Afterword

I hope you've found this book helpful. If you want to learn more about the research on which this book is based, visit the Blood Sugar 101 website at **http://www.bloodsugar101.com** or read the book, *Blood Sugar 101: What They Don't Tell You About Diabetes.*

You can learn more about low carbohydrate diets in my book, *Diet 101: The Truth About Low Carb Diets*. That book presents detailed information on the large, conclusive studies that have made clearer the strengths and weaknesses of this kind of diet and goes more deeply into the strategies that will make a low carb diet work.

If you find this book useful, please consider posting a review on the online website where you bought it. Positive reviews will make it easier for people who need this kind of information to find it.

And finally, when you have that appointment with your doctor where you're told your blood sugar has dropped dramatically, explain what you did to make it happen. The more of us they see who achieve normal blood sugars and with them normal health, the more likely they are to realize that maybe we're onto something.

Index

CPSIA information can be obtained
at www.ICGtesting.com
Printed in the USA
BVOW03s2236290817
492857BV00007B/81/P